# FORKING WELLNESS

# FORKING WELLNESS

Sophie Bertrand
MSc RNutr

Bari Stricoff
MSc RDN

From nutrition professionals and co-hosts of the podcast, **"Forking Wellness"**

**Your No-Nonsense Guide to Health and Nutrition**

MEYER & MEYER

British Library of Cataloguing in Publication Data
A catalogue record for this book is available from the British Library

**Forking Wellness**

Maidenhead: Meyer & Meyer Sport (UK) Ltd., 2021
ISBN: 978-1-78255-209-3

Aachen, Auckland, Beirut, Cairo, Cape Town, Dubai, Hägendorf, Hong Kong, Indianapolis, Maidenhead, Manila, New Delhi, Singapore, Sydney, Tehran, Vienna

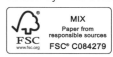 Member of the World Sport Publishers' Association (WSPA), www.w-s-p-a.org
Printed by Print Consult GmbH, Munich, Germany

ISBN: 978-1-78255-209-3
Email: info@m-m-sports.com
www.thesportspublisher.com

# Contents

# About Us and
# Our Story

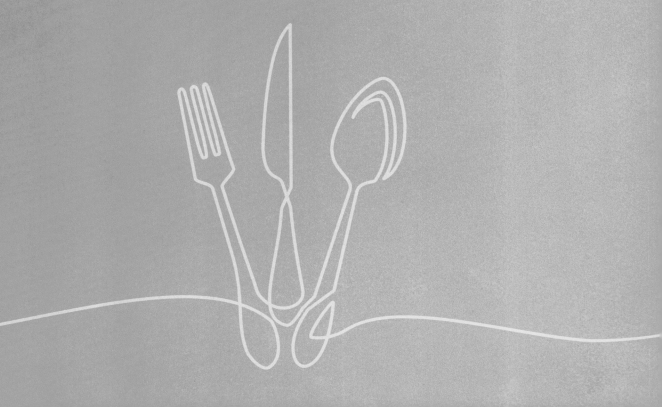

# About Sophie

When I was growing up, you might have found reason to call me the fussiest eater in the world. In fact, up until about the age of 14, my diet was largely made up of plain, beige foods (i.e. chicken, chips [aka fries], and bread). But I could always count on my mum to serve me broccoli and carrots at dinnertime. My plain diet wasn't deliberate—I just didn't find food that exciting, and I had no interest in trying new things. I'd never really been aware of or bothered by my body, but that all changed at the age of 14, when the size 0, skinny-model look seemed like the only acceptable body type, and I started to look at my body differently. Although I wasn't and never had been 'fat', that became what I saw when I looked in the mirror, so I began pursuing behaviours I believed would help me achieve the perfect body. I could write a whole book on my story alone, but I'll try and keep it brief. By the age of 17, after three years of

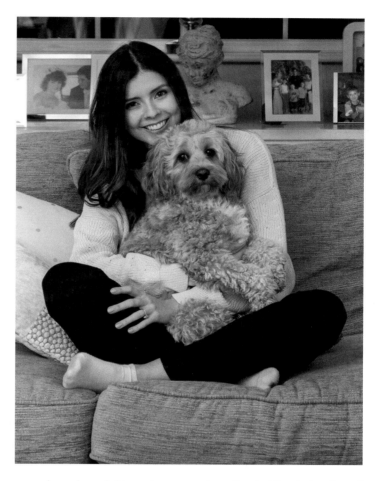

dedicating my life to weight loss, I was severely underweight, and my parents noticed. After being forced to commit to four months of intense therapy, by the age of 18 I was a 'normal' weight again—but still hugely dissatisfied with my body. So I decided I wouldn't lose *as* much weight as I did last time, and I was confident I could find a balance between eating what I thought was healthy and staying thin enough to be happy with my body. Well, let me tell you—that balance doesn't exist.

I had always been a perfectionist, a high achiever, and pretty controlling. But as I came to the end of my teenage years, I questioned what might happen if I put all that energy into something different—something that meant I wouldn't be obsessing over my food and body every day. Because the truth was, no number on the scales or reflection in the mirror was ever good enough for me. Having left school at 16 to pursue a diploma in fashion and design, I had no A levels. At the age of 20 I made the decision to go back to full-time education, and having not done A levels, I enrolled to do a foundation degree in psychology at Regent's University London and a year later was offered an academic scholarship. Four years later, I had a BSc in psychology under my belt and was a lot healthier (physically and mentally). Although my relationship with food wasn't what you'd consider normal, it was better than it had been, and I'd even tried (and liked) new foods. I remember that two weeks before we had exams I'd put myself on a brain-health diet, eating foods associated with enhanced cognitive function. So, from having no interest in food and health, throughout those four years I'd actually started to look at food in a different way and understand that important functions in the body needed a variety of foods to work. I decided I wanted to blog about this, so I grew more creative in the kitchen and decided to get on Instagram to post my recipes. As I developed more of an interest in food and well-being, I considered where my degree might take me. After finishing my university degree, I set off on a three-month trip with my sister (my favourite person in the world) to the West Coast of America. The rest of my family (my mum, dad, and two brothers) hired an RV for us all to do a trip of a lifetime, and then my sister and I stayed in LA for the rest of the three months. For the three weeks we were travelling in the RV, I ate to energise myself, to feel good, and because I enjoyed it. Being in a completely different environment was a real turning point for me, and it allowed me to fully enjoy the trip of my dreams. One day in West Hollywood, I was sitting in a health café and suddenly said, 'I want to be a nutritionist.' My sister was like, 'Cool, you should go for it'. She has always been incredibly supportive. At that point, I was convinced that clean eating was the only way to be healthy, and I wanted to learn more about the science behind how and what we eat. Looking back, I can say with confidence that now I know I was suffering from orthorexia.

As soon as I got home, I spent hours googling how I could go about my mission to become a registered nutritionist in the quickest way possible. But let me tell you this, qualifications aren't achieved overnight. I soon realised that if I wanted to be a registered nutritionist and take the role seriously, I was going to have to go back to full-time further education. I thought I'd regret not going for it, so I got in touch with the governing body for nutrition in the UK and enrolled on every single accredited CPD (continuing professional development) course they recommended. A year later, I was accepted to UCL (University College London) to study a master's in eating disorders and clinical nutrition, and I couldn't have been more excited. The summer before I started, I went back to the US with my sister for three months, but weeks before I left for the trip, I met the love of my life, Ash. After not seeing him for three months, I came back from the best trip of my life, and two months later, he moved down from Manchester, and I moved out of my rented flat in London, back to my parents' house so he and I could save for our own place. One evening we sat and, between us, ate a whole box of chocolates (something we now do often!). I remember thinking how even a year before that I'd have felt very guilty, but I didn't that night. I was so incredibly happy in life, it didn't even bother me.

When I started my master's, I realised I definitely didn't know as much about nutrition as I thought I did. It was the toughest year of my life, and I was working part-time and couldn't keep up with the amount of information there was to take in. Long days, weekends dedicated to studying, countless assignments, sporadic exams, hospital placements, and a lot of breakdowns later—I'd qualified as a nutritionist. And met Bari.

After finishing my studies, I reached out to (you could say *stalked*) my wonderful friend and mentor Rhiannon Lambert, desperate for her to give me work experience and train me on how to work with clients—something you're not taught in a degree programme. My persistence worked, and she hired me three months later to work for her company Rhitrition. Still building my Instagram page, I decided to turn what I called *Sophie's Healthy Kitchen* into a business. I was doing my best to build it alongside working with Rhiannon, but nine months later, I decided to take the plunge and go at my own business full-time, whilst still seeing clients at Rhitrition on a freelance basis. I emailed companies I wanted to work with, attended events, and networked as much as I could to start bringing in enough work to support my own business. I have to say, I couldn't have done any of this without Ash, who supported the both of us whilst I found my feet, and we managed to buy our first property, where we now live with our gorgeous cavapoo, Bear. Now, as well as successfully running my own business, I see clients at Rhitrition, and Rhiannon (RNutr) remains a treasured friend and mentor with regard to my nutrition work.

Having had such an unhealthy relationship with food growing up, I've realised that being happy within yourself is more important than obsessing over trying to be the 'perfect' version of healthy, and in my eyes, all food is fit. We're all just trying to make the most of our lives, and seeing food as an enemy makes everything more difficult. You can have your brownies, chocolate, and ice cream, and you can also have your buddha bowls, greens, and casseroles—food should be about enjoyment as well as supporting your overall health. And what fun is it eating only what we think we *should* be eating? No fun at all!

# About Bari

For anyone who knew me as a child, my career choice comes as no surprise. I'm from a family of foodies. My grandfather is a true culinary pioneer and the only Jew from Brooklyn who can whip up an authentic Szechuan feast you wouldn't believe. (The man can work miracles with some fresh garlic, ginger, and his cleverness.) But everything I know (both the good and the bad), I learned from my mother, Fran. I can honestly say I want to grow up to be just like her. Besides being extremely charismatic and tenacious, Fran (better known as Franny) is a classically trained chef—and a pretty good one, if I must admit (being biased, of course). While most kids were off playing sports or hanging with their friends

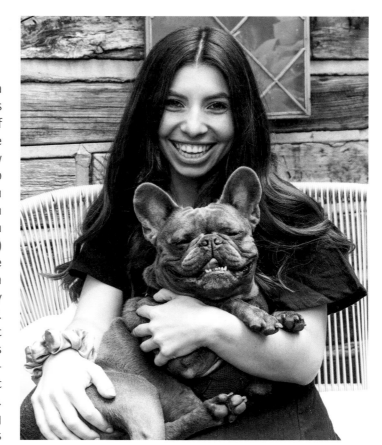

on weekends, I was begging my mom to let me come to work with her. She even bought me my own matching chef coat when I was eight, my favourite gift to date. I'd stand on milk crates to chop vegetables, roll meatballs, and peel potatoes. My love for food and cooking started at a young age, which led to my eclectic palate. Not all 10-year-olds would opt for raw scallops or periwinkle snails over chicken nuggets.

Although I had a burning passion for food and a love for cooking, I was also an extremely self-conscious teenager and highly judgmental of my appearance. I knew I wanted to be healthy and always tried to be the best version of myself, but I didn't quite understand what good nutrition was and what *healthy* truly meant. (Does anyone?) So, to learn more about portion control and how to make healthy choices, I began Weight Watchers at the ripe old age of 12 years old, with a signed doctor's note that I wasn't to lose any weight. I'd sit in on the weekly meetings and listen to older men and women complain about their food, weight, and lack of willpower.

Instead of helping me better understand food and nutrition, my exposure to Weight Watchers instilled rigid habits and initiated my poor relationship with food. I feared Caesar salad and found comfort in the fact that three Hershey's KISSES were worth only one point. That poor relationship with food continued until I graduated high school. But at my core I knew this wasn't healthy, nor was it how I wished to continue. So, with my passion for food and my interest in health and nutrition, complemented by a knack for the biological sciences, I applied to college (university), with the hope of majoring in dietetics and in finally learning from a scientific perspective how to be healthy.

Spoiler alert: it took me four years after graduating university to truly understand what healthy means.

In 2011, I enrolled on the University of Delaware Honors Program's dietetics programme. And much to my surprise, a degree in dietetics meant multiple semesters of biology, chemistry, biochemistry, organic chemistry, microbiology, and pathophysiology. But, four (long) years later, I graduated with a degree in dietetics, a minor in psychology, and a certificate of business essentials. But my journey to becoming a registered dietitian didn't stop there. I moved back home to Long Island to complete my dietetics internship, which consisted of more than 1200 hours of supervised practice in the clinical, foodservice, and community sectors. I was working for a private-practice dietitian, helping people lower their cholesterol, manage their diabetes, and control their Irritable Bowel Syndrome (IBS) symptoms. But while I had all the necessary skills to help them understand their conditions and educate them on the foods they should and shouldn't be eating, it became increasingly evident that there was a huge gap in my nutrition education—I had minimal training on understanding why they chose to eat foods they knew were harmful to their health. In other words, I wasn't a psychologist. But I quickly realised that psychological principles remain fundamental to achieving any lifestyle change, especially when it comes to changing your food habits.

When I completed my dietetics internship, passed the national exam, and finally earned those three letters after my name, RDN (registered dietitian nutritionist), I knew my educational journey remained incomplete. At the time, I had been in a long-distance relationship for three years with my boyfriend, Mark, who lived just outside London. Naturally, I enrolled on a master's programme in eating disorders and clinical nutrition at University College London, to combine my dietetics degree with a better understanding of psychology, while simultaneously uniting my professional and personal trajectories. So, I packed my bags (two 50 lb. suitcases, to be exact) and moved to the land of tea, biscuits, and fish and chips.

For the next year and a bit, I was a slave to this master's programme. The first half wasn't too bad as it was a natural extension of my dietetics background. But the psychology and eating-disorders modules tested my limits – they were bloody hard. But they were also extremely interesting and enjoyable. Plus, as Sophie mentioned, that's when our friendship began!

> To be honest, I coerced Sophie into taking a shot of tequila with me at the local pub after finishing our first exam. We had just become friends, and I'm 100 percent certain she obliged only due to being painfully polite (which is very British) and that it was the last shot of tequila she'll ever have, ha ha.

But when I finally finished six years of higher education, the reality of being an adult quickly set in. I was a 24-year-old registered dietitian with an MSc from one of the world's best universities, and I had no idea how to make my career goals come true. I wanted to stay in the UK with Mark and work as a registered dietitian. But sadly, that wasn't feasible as my reality was an imminently expiring visa and a *fork* ton of student debt.

For the next two years, my life was anything but stable. I split my time between New York and London to satisfy all my legal and visa restrictions, which meant I was unable to hold a steady job in any one location for long. So, I decided to embrace my entrepreneurial spirit and work for myself. I turned my hobby of an Instagram—@travelingdietitian—into a business—@barithedietitian. I worked with private clients via a telehealth platform to deliver digital nutrition services and worked with brands to develop recipes for social media, while building a blog. On the outside, life looked great. I was travelling to and from Europe and working for myself in my mid-20s. But in reality, I was suffering from crippling anxiety, stress, and loneliness. This soon manifested in extremely high cortisol levels (a stress hormone we'll discuss later) and subsequent alopecia. Having my hair fall out was a huge wake-up call for me. As someone who dedicated her life to helping others improve their health, how had I let mine suffer so much? In that moment, I grasped the importance of a more holistic approach to health and nutrition. I could eat all the kale and wild salmon I could find, but if I wasn't looking after both my body and my mind, I wasn't living a healthy lifestyle. (More of this to come throughout the book.)

Following this realisation, I truly committed everything I could to ensuring I was both happy and healthy. After an extremely intense visa application process, I finally landed back in the UK on a more permanent basis, back with Mark and back with Oscar (our puppy). I learned that while I loved working for myself and having the creative outlet it gave me, it wasn't bringing me joy. I wanted to have a bigger impact, work with more individuals, meet new people, and implement some much-needed structure and stability in my life.

Enter Second Nature, the London health-tech start-up where I found career bliss. Dedicated to helping people optimise their health, Second Nature also takes a holistic approach towards a healthy lifestyle. Here I can help hundreds of individuals a week build healthier habits, shift their mindset, improve their confidence, and lower their risk for chronic illness. I'm forever grateful to Second Nature for helping me develop as a dietitian and teaching me what it takes to build a successful company.

So, throughout the last 15 years, I've learned *a lot*, both personally and professionally. I've learned the number on the scale doesn't define your health nor your happiness. I've learned to focus on the things I can add to my life, not take away. I've learned the importance of stress management, quality sleep, and a reusable water bottle. But most importantly, I've learned how to appropriately define *health and wellness*, a unique concept on which Sophie and I feel passionate about educating others!

# How We Came Together

It's funny how two people from opposite sides of the world can have so much in common. While we met during our master's degrees at University College London, our friendship evolved beyond the classroom. Sure, we first bonded over where we wanted to eat in between lectures, but we soon realised we shared much more in common than our lunch orders. We both had our own food blogs, loved to develop recipes, shared a non-diet approach to health and nutrition, had struggled in the past with our own relationship with food, and were ultimately passionate about helping others.

When I (Bari) came back to the UK for the second time, after being in America for five months, Sophie and I made plans to catch up. Of course, this entailed getting together (with the dogs) to cook a delicious recipe to share with our followers. But what transpired from that day was special. We both felt there was a gap in the nutrition space. There were the nutrition professionals who were fanatical about a single cause or area of research, such as digestive health, longevity, or plant-based nutrition. There were the nutrition bloggers without any qualifications spreading misinformation about things like celery juice (sigh). There were also the public-health nutrition professions, relaying the guidelines and stating the foods we should eat, the foods we should limit, and how to be 'healthy'—while continuing to remain neutral in their opinions. There were the body-positive, non-diet activists, who were doing incredible things to break down stigmas and fight against diet culture.

And then there was us—somewhere in the middle.

> What does it forking mean to be perfect anyway? If you ask us, it sounds boring.

We don't live in a black-and-white world, so why should we have to label ourselves as a certain type of nutritionist or dietitian? If we had to put a label on ourselves, it would be something like 'We're anti-diet health professionals who strive for balance in all aspects of life. We like salads and avocados. We eat chocolate and crisps (chips). Sometimes we work out, and sometimes we'd rather be lazy. We're not perfect—nor do we try to be. We don't want to pigeonhole ourselves into a single area of nutrition but want to show people how to really live a healthy and balanced life with no sacrifices or food obsessions. We know there's no one-size-fits-all approach, and we have a judgment-free policy. We understand the science, but we also understand that science doesn't always fit into everyday situations. But we're not just a registered nutritionist and a registered dietitian. We're real people. And we don't need a forking label.

So, we sat on the couch in Sophie's house, and she looked at me and said, 'We should start a podcast'. Genius. What a fitting way to discuss our thoughts and opinions in an easy-to-digest manner. We can articulate the research and give an honest, relatable account of how to apply it to everyday life. And voilà—*Forking Wellness* was born. Because let's be honest—what the fork is wellness?

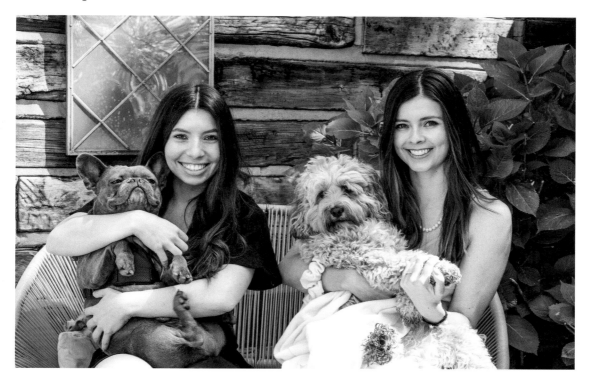

# Our Philosophy

## WHAT WE WANT TO ACHIEVE

With the success of our podcast—and the community that formed around it—came the idea for this book.

It's hard to put into words what we want to achieve, because it also sounds like common sense. With all the confusing information out there, we simply want to streamline the concept of *'wellness'*. We know the word *wellness* is extremely vague and ambiguous, but bear with us as we attempt to show you what it truly means. We're not going to tell you how much or what to eat or how to live your life but rather give you the tools and education to come to that decision for yourself. And what your wellness looks like will undoubtedly differ from everyone else's.

Science can be daunting, but it depends on how you interpret it. Traditionally, it starts with a question or thought. Then you form a hypothesis, which leads to an experiment and eventually a conclusion, which is then translated to the masses. It seems black-and-white. I mean, your experiment either proves or disproves your hypothesis, right?

Wrong.

These news headlines are often fictional but are representative of feasible newspaper articles.

On any given day, multiple conflicting research papers could be published. For example, one may read 'Low-Fat Diets Linked to Improved Cardiovascular Health' while others claim, 'Scientist No Longer Believe Saturated Fat Causes Heart Disease', 'Unsaturated Fats Protect Against Cardiovascular Disease', and 'The Keto Diet Is Linked to Longevity'. Like, what the fork?

So what do we actually take away from those headlines?

If I restrict my fat intake, I can improve my cardiovascular health. But not all fat—because unsaturated fat, like olive oil, is protective against heart disease. And saturated fat, like animal products, may not be the cause of heart disease. So why am I limiting my fat? And if high-fat diets, like keto, are linked to longevity, should I become keto? But the first headline said to reduce my total fat for heart health. What the fork?

Throughout this book, we want to help you feel empowered, not confused. Most of the time, science exists in a vacuum, and to mimic those outcomes, you must live a pretty restrictive and rigid lifestyle. Not only is this unsustainable, but it fosters an unhealthy relationship with food (another concept we'll discuss later in the book).

But, at the end of the day, science is amazing, and nutritional science is exciting—or at least *we* think so. We promise to break everything down into something easy to digest and to help you understand how to practically integrate healthy habits into your overall lifestyle without labels or restrictions. We want to open your mind to a broader definition of *wellness* that's not solely defined by the food on your plate but is a more holistic approach that encompasses your mental and physical well-being.

If you've ever felt confused about what to eat, this book is for you.

If you've ever felt conflicted about how to achieve optimum health but remain sane and enjoy the foods you love at the time, this book is for you.

If you've ever wanted to ditch the diets and the labels but feared what would happen next, this book is for you.

If you want to learn how to eat mindfully, this book is for you.

If you want to fall in love with food again and feel confident in the kitchen, this book is for you.

If you want to learn what realistic wellness is—you guessed it—this book is for you.

## NOT YOUR AVERAGE NUTRITION BOOK

If you're looking for a list of things to do followed by a list of things to abstain from, you're reading the wrong book. There are no good-food or bad-food lists, no 'healthy swaps', no rules, and no restrictions. There are no meal plans, no guidelines for calories, and no false promises.

But let's be honest, everything we just mentioned is the reason why diets don't work. We promise to elaborate on this further throughout the book and provide the facts to back it up, but for now, picture this:

You pick up a new diet book, read it front to back, and internalise all the information. You cut out sugar, dairy, carbs, fat, and alcohol. Essentially, you're living off salad with grilled chicken and no dressing. (How boring!) But you lose weight, and you feel 'better'. So now what? It worked. What happens next? Did you learn any valuable lessons on nutrition or incorporate any healthy habits into your routine? Did you deal with any emotional attachments you have with food?

Probably not.

You'll most likely resort to your previous eating habits, leaving you feeling down and defeated. But not to worry, you can start a new diet with a new set of restrictions on Monday, right?

And so the diet cycling begins. And trust us, we've been there—it's not fun. But most importantly, it's not helpful, sustainable, or healthy.

So, unlike your average nutrition book, we want to show you what a truly balanced lifestyle looks like.

Nutrition is undoubtedly important, even integral to a healthy lifestyle. But, it's not absolute. And what even is *healthy*? It's such a vague and ambiguous term that means something different to all of us. While the food we eat has a big impact on our physical and mental health, there's so much more that needs to be considered, and it's going to look different for everyone.

Things like sleep, hydration, stress, and self-care also play a huge role in our overall health, which is something we want to emphasise. While we're both nutrition professionals, we believe that health encompasses so much more than the food you consume. It may seem ironic that a registered nutritionist and a registered dietitian aren't preaching about pursuing the perfect diet. We're preaching about finding a routine that works for you—one that encompasses balance and self-care, takes care of both your body and your mind, and is easy to stick with in the long run. We believe in no sacrifices and in realistic decisions.

We don't believe in focusing on every facet of nutrition, because, to be honest, it can be too overwhelming. You can devote your life to eating for longevity or optimising your gut health, but what things do you miss out on in the pursuit of perfection? We truly believe in making realistic choices that will benefit your overall health, both physical and mental. It's not about being perfect, it's about balance and happiness. Yes, we want to promote eating a diet rich in vegetables, but that doesn't mean you have to cut out crisps. And of course we want to educate you on the benefits of meal prepping, but that doesn't mean you have to be a slave to your kitchen. It's all about striking that balance.

We want everyone to be able to take away some helpful information from this book. We realise, even hope, that this book and our philosophy have a different impact on every reader. Even as best friends, our health decisions are completely different, as is what wellness is for each of us—as it all should be.

You shouldn't aspire to have someone else's wellness routine; you should aspire to find your own. Remember, we're all unique.

We hope this book inspires you to make healthier and more-balanced choices, whatever that may look like for you.

# Nutrition Basics

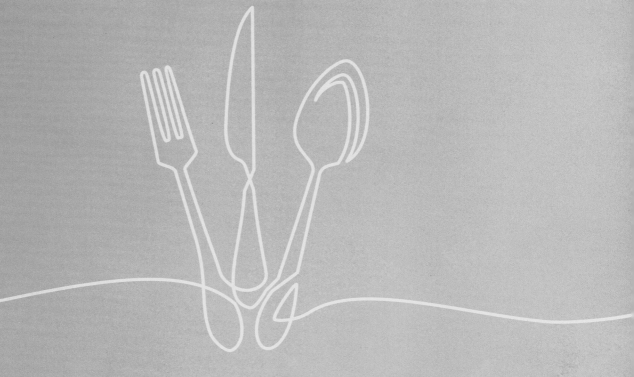

In this chapter we break down both macro- and micronutrients to explain the importance of each one. Feel free to skip ahead if you have a good understanding or foundation in nutrition.

# Macronutrients

Macronutrients are energy-providing nutrients that include carbohydrates, protein, and fat. They're needed in large quantities and helping the body with many different functions. We also discuss fibre, as it is fast becoming the most talked about nutrient.

## CARBOHYDRATES

Carbohydrates (or carbs) may be the most demonised food group, yet they have an important place in a well-balanced diet.

Carbs tend to be split into two categories: simple or 'free' sugars (e.g. sweets and fruit juices) and starchy (also known as complex) carbs (e.g. bread, rice, potatoes). Starchy carbs are often divided further into white and whole-grain carbs. We want to each fill our plate with more starchy carbs than simple sugars, but that doesn't mean they have to be eliminated.

All carbohydrates get converted to glucose, which can be used by your body and brain for energy. Lack of carbohydrates in your diet may result in low energy levels, both physically and mentally. If your brain doesn't have sufficient amounts of carbs to use, the body can convert fatty acids into energy to meet the brain's requirements. Whilst this adaptation is happening, the body has to break down protein for energy, which may result in muscle loss—so it's not the wisest move to limit your carbohydrate intake!

Carbohydrate-rich foods are also rich in many vitamins and minerals (a.k.a. micronutrients, which we'll discuss). Thus, when you eliminate or cut down on carbohydrates, you may also be missing out on other essential nutrients.

# FIBRE

Fibre was the unsung hero of nutrition for a long time. Only healthcare professionals seemed to realise how vital this nutrient was for regularity as well as cardiovascular disease. But with the recent rise in the microbiome and gut-health research, fibre has become the shining star of nutrients, which is well deserved.

Fibre is the nondigestible portion of the food item found in plants. There are two types of fibre: soluble and insoluble.

Soluble fibre dissolves in water to form a thick gel-like substance in the stomach and gets broken down by bacteria in the large intestine. Soluble fibre has been linked to improved cardiovascular health (e.g. Cheerios) by lowering LDL (bad) cholesterol. Soluble fibre also helps control blood-sugar levels by delaying the release of sugar into the blood.

Insoluble fibre doesn't dissolve in water and passes through the GI tract intact (undigested). Insoluble fibre has been shown to improve digestion and relieve constipation as it provides bulk for stool formation and speeds up the movement of food and waste through the digestive system.

Both types of fibre increase your feeling of fullness and improve the quality of gut microbiota. This improves digestion, mood, blood sugar, and more. High-fibre diets have also been shown to be protective against certain types of cancer, specifically bowel cancer.

As mentioned, fibre comes from plant sources, such as fruit, vegetables, legumes, nuts, seeds, whole grains, and wheat bran. The following are some common sources of fibre:

» avocado: 6.7 g fibre per 100 g

» raspberries: 6.5 g fibre per 100 g

» artichokes: 8.6 g fibre per 100 g

» lentils: 7.9 g fibre per 100 g

» chickpeas: 7.6 g fibre per 100 g

» oats: 10.6 g fibre per 100 g

» almonds: 12.5 g fibre per 100 g

Other foods that are good sources of fibre include apples, split peas, brussels sprouts, chia seeds, sweet potatoes, popcorn, beetroots (beets), and carrots.

The average person consumes about only 14 grams per day, while the recommendation is 25–35 grams per day (Harvard, n.d.). This below-average consumption has resulted in a big public-health push to raise awareness for the importance of fibre consumption.

*Top Tips*

**Try these to increase your fibre intake:**

» **Increase your fruit and vegetable intake. Choose whole fruits over fruit juices.**

» **Aim for three servings of whole grains a day, such as porridge (aka oatmeal) at breakfast, whole-wheat bread at lunch, and brown rice at dinner.**

» **Be mindful of refined grains and products made with refined grains, which can be high in added sugars, saturated fat, and sodium (e.g. cakes, crisps, cookies, biscuits).**

» **Consider fruit (especially berries) as a part of your daily snacks.**

» **Add beans or lentils to salads, soups, and side dishes.**

**If you're not used to eating high-fibre foods regularly, make changes gradually to avoid problems with gas and diarrhoea. Drink plenty of water to minimise intestinal upset.**

## PROTEIN

Protein is extremely important for building and repairing body tissue. Protein is used to make hormones and enzymes and are essential for building muscles, cartilage, bones, skin, and blood cells.

Amino acids are the building blocks that make up protein, and essential amino acids must be derived from food as they can't be made by the body (unlike non-essential amino acids). A complete protein is one that contains all the essential amino acids. Animal proteins are complete proteins and include meat, poultry, fish, eggs, and dairy. There are also a few non-animal complete proteins: soya, hempseed, quinoa, and buckwheat, however, some plant-based proteins can be paired together in order to assemble complete proteins:

» red beans and rice

» black beans and polenta

» hummus and seed crackers

» chickpeas and quinoa

» peanut butter and whole-grain bread

The reference nutrient intake (RNI) for adults is set at 0.75 g of protein per day per kilogram of body weight, however, the amount of protein one's body needs may change during **a person's** lifetime. The ideal amount of protein for any one individual tends to depend on a variety of factors, including age, muscle mass, activity level, and overall health. If you have a physically demanding job or are particularly active every day, your body may require more protein than the daily recommendation. Additionally, older adults tend to have increased protein needs, which may be up to 50 percent higher than the RNI, the recommended daily amount (Morais, Chevalier, and Gougeon 2006) as it may help prevent sarcopenia—reduction in muscle mass—and osteoporosis—weakening of the bones (Gaffney-Stomberg et al. 2009).

## PROTEIN SUPPLEMENTS

Protein powders have become very popular in the last few years, and there tend to be mixed opinions about whether or not we should or need to be using them. We don't actually need protein powder, and if you're eating a varied and well-balanced diet that includes chicken, fish, tofu, eggs, yoghurt, pulses, and so forth, you're probably meeting your daily requirement. But protein powders can be a great option if you feel you need to add a bit more protein to your diet. For instance, if you're on the go a lot and need something quick to grab and go, a protein smoothie may be the way forward. Unfortunately, there are a lot of protein powders on the market that have added sugars or artificial sweeteners, and if you're consuming protein powder regularly, it's a good idea to find one that you enjoy that isn't packed with too many additional ingredients.

## FAT

Fat has important roles to play in a person's diet, including carrying fat-soluble vitamins (Donovan 2018). There are many different types of fats, so we're going to break it down a little further for you.

There are two groups of fats: saturated and unsaturated. Unsaturated fats include polyunsaturated or monounsaturated fats.

Saturated fats are usually found in animal products (fatty meats, butter, cheese, cream etc.) and can also be found in shop-bought cakes and pastries. Saturated fats are often considered less healthy than other fats as there's some research linking them to an increased risk of heart disease and raised cholesterol levels. But this isn't to say they can't be included in a well-balanced diet.

Unsaturated fats tend to be present more in plant-based foods, such as nuts, seeds, and avocados.

We need fat in our diet, but the quantity in which we consume it and the quality of the fat does carry some importance. It's suggested that around one-third of our energy intake should come from fat, preferably more unsaturated than saturated. Many people don't include enough fat in their diet, particularly essential fatty acids, often referred to as omega-3s.

## OMEGA-3S

Omega-3 fatty acids, also known as polyunsaturated fatty acids (PUFAs), are considered to be essential fatty acids, meaning we can't synthesise them within the body and must get them from food. Omega-3s help improve heart health by reducing plaque in the arteries and decreasing triglycerides in the blood. Omega-3s have also been shown to decrease inflammation, improve immunity, support the endocrine system, and aid in cognition.

There are three types of omega-3s: ALA, DHA, and EPA. ALAs are found in oils of plants, such as soya beans, flaxseeds, chia seeds, and walnuts. DHAs and EPAs are found in fatty fish, such as salmon, mackerel, and albacore tuna. Our bodies must convert ALAs into EPAs and then into DHAs in order to absorb it into the body. But humans aren't great at this conversion, since we convert only about 15 percent. Thus, the body much prefers consuming EPA and DHA sources, in order to reap the benefits of omega-3s. In fact, the American Heart Association recommends consuming fatty fish (100 g serving) at least twice a week (Mayo 2014), while the NHS recommends consuming it at least once a week (2018).

# Micronutrients

Macronutrients include vitamins and minerals that, unlike macronutrients, are needed in small amounts. They're essential for normal functioning of the body.

## FAT-SOLUBLE VITAMINS

As stated in the name, fat-soluble vitamins can be absorbed into the body only in the presence of fat. Additionally, our bodies store these vitamins (especially vitamins A and E) within our body tissue.

**Vitamin A:** Most commonly known to help support vision, vitamin A is also important for maintaining healthy bones, teeth, skin, and cellular membranes. Foods rich in vitamin A tend to be colourful, such as yellow fruit, orange fruit, and dark, leafy green vegetables.

**Vitamin D:** We get most of our vitamin D from the sun as our bodies aren't very efficient at converting vitamin D from food into vitamin D the body can use. But as most people's sun exposure is inconsistent throughout the year, there are several public-health initiatives aimed at increasing our vitamin D in the winter months. Additionally, many foods are fortified with vitamin D, and natural forms can be found in egg yolks and oily fish. Vitamin D is essential for healthy bones, teeth, and muscles.

**Vitamin E:** Vitamin E acts as an antioxidant in the body, protecting against free radicals and cellular damage in addition to supporting the immune system. Vitamin E is best found in whole grains, nuts, vegetable oil, and green vegetables.

**Vitamin K:** Vitamin K is a very interesting vitamin as it's not only found in certain foods, such as leafy, green vegetables, but the bacteria in your gut actually synthesise vitamin K in the large intestine. Vitamin K is necessary to aid in blood clotting.

## WATER-SOLUBLE VITAMINS

Unlike fat-soluble vitamins, water-soluble vitamins are readily absorbed into the body regardless of dietary fat being present. But water-soluble vitamins aren't stored within the body, so any vitamins that remain unused are then excreted. Water-soluble vitamins consist of the B complex and vitamin C.

**Thiamine (vitamin B1):** Thiamine is needed to convert food into energy and to maintain proper nervous-system functions and metabolic processes, such as immunity. Thiamine can be readily found in pork, legumes, and peas and is often fortified in wheat products, such as cereals, bread, and pasta.

**Riboflavin (vitamin B2):** Riboflavin is also needed to convert food into energy and aid in the production of red blood cells. Found in liver, eggs, dark, leafy green vegetables, legumes, grains, and milk, riboflavin is often destroyed by UV light, so it's important to make sure your milk is stored in an opaque jar.

**Niacin (vitamin B3):** Just like vitamins B1 and B2, niacin is important for energy production, the nervous system, digestive health, and enzyme functions. Niacin is mainly found in meat, poultry, fish, whole grains, and vegetables.

**Pyridoxine (vitamin B6):** Pyridoxine is a very important vitamin as it plays a key role in red-blood-cell production as well as amino-acid metabolism. Thus, as your protein intake increases, your vitamin B6 requirements also increase. Pyridoxine is found in an abundance of foods, such as meat, poultry, fish, wheat, and ready-to-eat cereals.

**Folate (folic acid):** Most commonly known for being an essential nutrient during pregnancy, folic acid is important for preventing neural-tube defects in newborns. Additionally, folic acid is imperative for DNA and red-blood-cell synthesis. As a public-health measure to prevent neural-tube defects, folic acid is fortified to most cereals. Other sources include leafy green vegetables, legumes and citrus.

**Vitamin B12:** Exclusively found in animal products, vitamin B12 is important for new cell production and nerve functions. Vitamin-B12 deficiency is common in long-time vegans and vegetarians, however, many foods are now fortified with vitamin B12, including many plant-based milks. Other sources include meat, eggs, dairy, poultry, and seafood.

**Biotin:** Essential for the production of fatty acids, biotin is also part of an enzyme needed for energy metabolism. It's found mainly in eggs, wheat, liver, bananas, salmon, and dairy products.

**Pantothenic acid:** Pantothenic acid is actually part of an enzyme that's used in the energy breakdown process, which helps convert food into energy. Pantothenic acid is widely abundant in most foods.

**Vitamin C:** Vitamin C acts as an antioxidant, protecting the body from cellular damage and free radicals. Vitamin C is also needed to produce collagen, a structural protein, and is vital in wound healing. Unlike other vitamins, vitamin C is primarily found in fruit and vegetables, especially citrus. Other sources include potatoes, dark green vegetables, yellow vegetables, and papayas.

## MINERALS

**Calcium:** Calcium is an essential mineral for building and maintaining strong bones and teeth and is regulated by the parathyroid hormone and vitamin D. It's also needed for muscle contraction, cardiac functioning, and nerve transmission. Calcium can be found in milk, cheese, yoghurt, beans, almonds, tofu, and leafy greens. You can now find foods that are fortified with calcium too.

**Phosphorus:** Phosphorus aids in the formation of bones and teeth and is needed to make protein for the growth, maintenance, and repair of cells. Phosphorus is found in meats, dairy, eggs, nuts, seeds, and whole grains.

**Iron:** Iron transfers oxygen from the lungs to tissue in the body and comes in two forms: heme and nonheme. Heme iron is easily absorbed by the body and can be found in meat and fish. Nonheme iron can be found in nuts, seeds, and leafy greens but isn't as bioavailable to the body as heme is. You can enhance absorption by pairing nonheme iron foods with foods rich in vitamin C.

**Magnesium:** Magnesium is needed to help maintain nerve and muscle function, strong bones, and a healthy immune system. It also aids in the production of energy and regulates sleep. Sources include nuts and seeds, leafy greens, fish, and fruits such as figs, bananas, and avocados.

**Zinc:** Zinc plays a role in cell division, growth, and wound healing. It also aids in the breakdown of carbohydrates. You can find zinc in meat, eggs, dairy products, nuts, and whole grains.

**Iodine:** Iodine supports the thyroid, which helps control metabolism. Found in fish and dairy products, it may need to be supplemented for those following a vegan diet.

**Manganese:** Manganese plays a role in energy metabolism, bone formation, and reducing inflammation. It can be found in nuts, beans, whole grains, and leafy greens.

**Copper:** This mineral is found in all body tissue, helping to maintain nerve cells and make red blood cells. It helps the body absorb iron and can be found in shellfish, nuts, seeds, leafy greens, and dark chocolate.

**Selenium:** The body needs small amounts of selenium to help make antioxidant enzymes that aid in preventing cell damage. Brazil nuts are one of the best sources, but selenium can also be found in meat and whole grains.

# Nutrient Diversity

Eating a variety of foods can help improve general well-being. Research suggests that adding more diversity to your diet and eating a variety of different foods from all food groups may reduce the risk of various health conditions, such as heart disease, stroke, some cancers, diabetes, and osteoporosis (Jackson and Collins 2014).

As humans, we're often creatures of habit, choosing to eat the same few foods on rotation. But when we eat the same food every day, we're receiving the same nutrients, from the same foods, in the same quantities. Thus, mixing up our food choices ensures we meet all our nutritional requirements, and consuming a more diversified and broader range of foods allows for more-extensive exposure to various dietary components and essential nutrients. Diversity in the diet also helps promote diversity within the gut, which has a great impact on our overall health, digestive health, immunity, blood-sugar balance, and more. (This is a more complex area that requires a whole separate book.)

Now, we know what you might be thinking—sounds expensive! There are often misconceptions around being healthy, including that it costs more money. But why does it have to be all or nothing? We're confident when we say eating a varied diet within a budget is possible—you just need to get savvy. Think tinned foods, frozen foods, and pantry staples. We guide you through getting savvy in the kitchen on page 99.

# Breaking Down
the Science

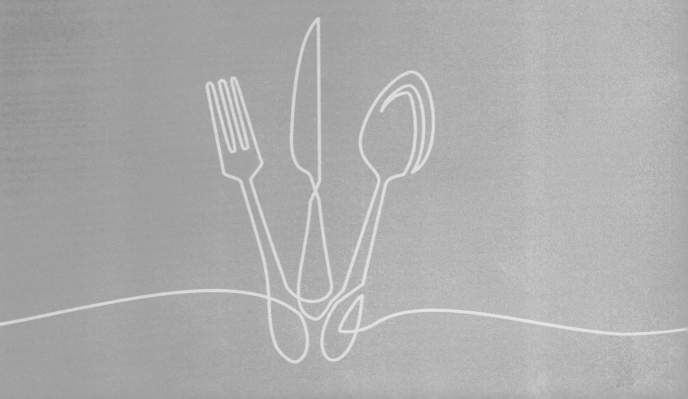

# Why Is Nutrition So Confusing?

In the words of Avril Lavigne, 'Why'd you have to go and make things so complicated?' Jokes aside, why does nutrition have to be so forking confusing? How can a single food be both good and bad for your health? And why do the guidelines and recommendations keep changing?

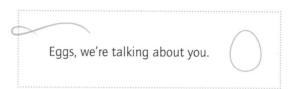

Eggs, we're talking about you.

## CURRENT RESEARCH

This section may seem a little more sciencey, but we think it's important to highlight the pitfalls of the current nutrition research.

Did you know the science of nutrition is relatively young? Scientific interest in the human body has existed for thousands of years, with the first human autopsy having been performed in 300 BC, by doctors in Alexandria (Kruszelnicki 2002). Here we are 2320 years later, and a lot has changed in our understanding of the human body (thanks to the evolution of man, education, and technology, of course). That's a pretty long time to be studying, evolving and updating our understanding of the human body. But it wasn't until 1926 (less than 100 years ago) that nutritional sciences began, with the identification of the first vitamin (Mozaffarian, Rosenberg, and Uauy 2018).

The first vitamin to be discovered was Vitamin C.

In the early 20th century, nutrition science consisted of discovering the macro- and micronutrients discussed in the previous chapter. Once these nutrients had all been discovered, the research shifted to focus on the specific amounts necessary to prevent deficiencies, such as scurvy, rickets, and beriberi. Eventually, these studies gave us the RDAs (recommended dietary allowances).

RDAs are the work of government-commissioned scientists paid to ascertain minimum dietary requirements in order to be prepared for war and were first released in 1941. These new guidelines for total calories and recommendations for things like total protein, calcium, and iron were first announced at the National Nutrition Conference on Defense in the US. How interesting!

But the research at this time focused on single nutrients and their effects on our overall health. In other words, this reductionist approach to nutrition led to the emphasis on fats (saturated vs. unsaturated) and carbohydrates (including sugar). Basically, the studies that were conducted around this time shamed single nutrients in relation to our health, essentially giving way to the rise of food phobias. Thankfully, in the last 20–30 years, our nutrition research has evolved, and we now have a more holistic understanding of overall health. Nonetheless, these early studies set the precedent for singling out certain nutrients or foods, which led to removing food types from one's diet in order to improve overall health.

But we're not saying all the research conducted was poor. In fact, it was these single-nutrient-focused studies that led to the conclusion that folic-acid deficiency during pregnancy results in neural-tube defects. These results eventually led to the fortification of folic acid in everyday foods and awareness for prenatal vitamins—very important advances in nutrition sciences (Sorkin et al. 2016).

Thankfully, the research studies conducted in more-recent years have focused less on single vitamins and minerals and more on the role of nutrition in overall health and noncommunicable chronic diseases (diabetes, cancers, cardiovascular disease, etc.). Although this is a step in the right direction, we want to briefly point out some of the pitfalls of nutrition research:

1. The gold-standard research studies are randomised controlled trials (RCTs), studies that best control for biases. Ideally, you want a double-blind RCT, which means neither the participants nor the scientists are aware of whether the participants are in the treatment or placebo group.

   In basic terms, there are very few well-controlled RCTs in the nutrition space. And the well-controlled studies we do have often consist of small sample sizes, making it difficult to generalise the information for the wider population (Weaver and Miller 2017).

2. It's very hard to perform studies on humans as there's so much interpersonal variability. In other words, we're all unique and have a different set of behaviours, family predispositions, lifestyle factors, genetics, gut microbiome, and much more. This makes it extremely difficult to make nutrition-related conclusions, which often leads us to use the average results of the study. But are every study's subjects diversified enough to represent the general population? Can we apply the conclusions to every race and ethnicity? Are the average conclusions accepted across all demographics and socioeconomic statuses?

3. Long-term data tends to be observational—to make many nutrition claims, we need to track behaviours over a long period of time. But these studies are non-experimental, which means we can conclude only correlation, not causation. For example, we may use observational research to say 'Consistent exercise for at least 150 minutes per week for five years is correlated with decreased risk of cardiovascular disease'. But we can't say, 'If you exercise for 150 minutes per week for five years, you won't suffer from cardiovascular disease' (Zhong et al. 2019).

   Unfortunately, much of the data from long-term observational studies is based on the recollection of food eaten or self-reported data (Archer, Pavela, and Lavie 2015). For example, the researcher may ask, 'How many servings of vegetables did you have every day over the last 10 years?' We can barely remember what we ate for dinner last night; how are we meant to accurately recall our eating patterns every day for the past 10 years? Alternatively, subjects may have to fill out a 24-hour food recall every specified number of days, months, or years. Again, these have proven to be highly inaccurate because we often overestimate the positives and underestimate the negatives. Clearly, this results in inaccurate data, which may lead to false nutrition claims (Zhong et al. 2019).

> If you're interested in reading more about the corruption of food companies within the research of nutrition, we recommend reading *Unsavory Truth: How Food Companies Skew the Science of What We Eat*, by Marion Nestle.

4. As governmental funds continue to dwindle, nutrition research studies are increasingly being funded by the private sector. And you guessed it—these studies have agendas. It's no secret that food companies will fund their own study in order to support the production and consumption of their products.

Now we're not here to dispute the claims made in the following studies, but we do want to shed light using a couple interesting examples.

Did you know that Mars has funded over 100 studies regarding the health benefits of chocolate and cocoa? Or that Coca-Cola funded a study concluding that sugar-sweetened beverages have no effects on your overall health or weight (Nestle 2001)?

Now don't get us wrong, we truly believe chocolate and soda can be part of an overall healthy lifestyle. But we're dubious of the research and stress the importance of an 'all foods are fit' mentality while we're not reiterating or citing the specific research conclusions.

In fact, a 2007 study, 'Relationship Between Funding Source and Conclusion Among Nutrition-Related Scientific Articles', concludes that industry funding led to biased conclusions in favour of the sponsors' products. Beyond food companies, this study suggests that even pharmaceutical companies can influence the research and whether a new clinical trial is conducted testing their drug (Lesser et al. 2007). (Shocking.)

Anyway, just remember that it's common for certain food companies to produce studies whose conclusions support the sale of their products.

5. And finally, many nutrition-related research studies fail to see the bigger picture. Most research studies are reductionistic in nature, as we mentioned previously. But we know good nutrition and overall health are affected by a multitude of variables. While

> Wellness is more than the food you eat. It also encompasses the lifestyle you live.

some studies attempt to control for things like family predispositions and exercise, very few control for other health factors such as sleep and stress management.

All of these factors are why nutrition is so forking confusing—because many of the studies are poorly controlled and are biased. That's why it's so important to read the original studies (not just the abstracts). But we know reading nutrition research papers isn't how most people want to spend their free time, which is completely understandable. Just take it as a PSA to proceed with caution when it comes to reading nutrition headlines, and if you're confused, always ask a qualified professional for guidance on nutrition information.

## TRENDS THROUGHOUT THE DECADES

It's comical to reflect back on the past century and see the evolution of dieting. Unfortunately, our society has, for decades, associated value, beauty, and self-worth with physical appearance, especially for women. And while we've seen a big shift in the 21st century with the rise of body positivity, body acceptance, and the intuitive-eating movements, our culture remains deeply rooted in the 'thin ideal'.

The 'thin ideal' refers to the concept that thin or slender women are the picture of beauty and that the epitome of beauty is defined by a flat stomach with slight curves. Picture Barbie. Who the fork looks like that?

We must admit that throughout the years diet trends have become more scientifically based, but that doesn't mean they're evidence based. It simply means the recommendations have gained some level of scientific or medical consciousness. Or you may wish to view this the other way: early diets were absolutely ludicrous and made no logical or scientific sense.

Let's start with the 1925 cigarette diet' (Really?) The Lucky Strike cigarette company launched a campaign capitalising on tobacco's appetite-suppressing quality Its 'Reach for a Lucky instead of a sweet' slogan urged consumers to smoke cigarettes to help shed the pounds (Serrur 2017). That sounds like a safe idea, but . . .

Instead of relying on other products, maybe you can pray the pounds away, thought Rev. Charlie Shedd. In 1957, the reverend published his book *Pray Your Weight Away*, in which he documented his weight-loss journey of more than 100 pounds, which he attributed to his newfound self-discipline, bestowed upon him as a result of prayer (Serrur 2017). And some think meditation is a bit woo-woo.

Or how about the 1970s sleeping-beauty diet, which encouraged individuals to simply go to sleep to avoid eating (Serrur 2017). The initial popularity of this diet coincided with the rise of sleeping pills, which meant people (mostly women) opted to use prescription drugs for the unintended purpose of weight loss. Although a good night's sleep has been linked to positive outcomes in terms of overall health and weight maintenance (a topic we'll later discuss), this wasn't the intention of the proponents. Instead, their message was interpreted as 'If you want to lose weight, don't eat. And you can't eat if you're sleeping, so if you feel hungry, pop a sleeping pill instead, and you'll wake up feeling lighter'. Urrggggg.

We believe these three diets each deserve their own paragraphs because of their outlandish nature and absence of any regard for health or nutrition. A big pet peeve we have with diets is how they focus on weight loss while ignoring the basic principles of health (or wellness).

So take a walk down memory lane with us as we document the other diet trends throughout history.

**1963:** Jean Nidetch founded Weight Watchers (now 'WW') in Queens, New York. What began as a group of women in her living room discussing how to best lose weight (Weight Watchers, n.d.) is now an international company worth over $160 million (more than £128 million). Based on a points system, Weight Watchers originally centred around low-fat meat and dairy and the omission of alcohol, sweets, and fatty foods. Each food was assigned a unique point value, and you had to stay below a certain number of points per day to lose weight. Essentially, the original plan was calorie counting that was covered in makeup.

**1969:** Across the pond, in Derbyshire, England, Margaret Miles-Bramwell founded Slimming World. Slimming World is a low-fat diet that encourages unlimited consumption of what the diet called *Syn-free* foods. The programme claims that no foods are off-limits, but each restricted food has a certain number of Syns attached. So if you have a piece of chocolate cake, are you a 'sinner'? We discuss later in the book how to build a healthy relationship with food.

**The 1970s:** The grapefruit diet claimed that having a serving of grapefruit with each meal would help you burn fat and lose weight (Serrur 2017). The original sample diet plan was low-calorie (1200 or fewer per day) and low-carbohydrate:

» Breakfast: ½ grapefruit, 2 eggs, and 2 slices bacon

» Lunch: ½ grapefruit, protein, and salad

» Dinner: ½ grapefruit, protein, and salad or vegetables

» Snack: 1 cup skimmed milk

**1975:** The Cookie Diet was created by Dr Sanford Siegal to help his patients control their hunger and lose weight. He claims his cookies (biscuits) are low-calorie and contain a 'special mixture of proteins that naturally suppress hunger' so you can stick to a low-calorie diet. During his weight-loss phase, his recommendation is to have nine cookies per day (one to two cookies every two hours) and then protein and vegetables for dinner (Cookie Diet, n.d.).

**1977:** SlimFast hit the market, promoting their high-protein and low-fat meal-replacement shakes to help people lose weight (SlimFast, n.d.).

**The 1980s:** The cabbage-soup diet, also known as the Dolly Parton diet, introduced its seven-day diet plan. The diet promoted unlimited consumption of its cabbage soup (basically, cabbage and water) along with a narrow list of other 'allowed' foods (Frey, n.d.).

**1985:** Jenny Craig entered the scene with her prepackaged, low-calorie meals and one-on-one support from what she called *consultants*. The qualifications and criteria required to become a consultant remain unknown. Basically, if you pay for the Jenny Craig meals and don't deviate from the provided food, you're promised to lose weight.

**The 1990s:** The low-fat craze was in full force! Based on some weak observational studies, the assumption that dietary fat and cholesterol increase the risk for cardiovascular disease led people to consume a low-fat diet to help prevent heart disease. Ironically, the rise of obesity rates in America directly correlates with the low-fat movement. Let's be very clear about this: correlation doesn't equal causation, but it's interesting, nonetheless.

**1998:** Remember Jared? Well, he claimed to lose weight by eating nothing but Subway, which inevitably led to the Subway diet. But this was another calorie-restriction diet, since he admitted to skipping breakfast and having no more than 1,200 calories (and of just Subway) per day. He also later admitted to including exercise in this routine (Davidson 2013).

**The early 2000s:** Low-carb diets became increasingly popular. Claiming to promote weight loss and to improve health, the Atkins diet book was released in 2003. Atkins (n.d.) was one of many low-carb diets that were highly restrictive and claimed you could lose weight quickly by cutting out all carbohydrates. We'll discuss this more in detail soon.

**The 2000s:** Juice cleanses claimed to help remove toxins from your body, promote weight loss, and improve overall health. Let's not forget that juice is just water, natural sugars, and a small number of vitamins and minerals. We also have kidneys and a liver that help us naturally detox. Another low-calorie fad diet that lacks any scientific evidence.

**Approximately 2010:** The baby-food diet was another overnight success (in terms of fad diets) for its ability to produce quick weight loss. But this is yet again another low-calorie diet that lacks overall diversity and makes meeting any nutrition requirements difficult. Remember, adults and infants have very different nutritional needs.

Thanks to the rise of Instagram, #cleaneating became a thing. A 2019 study defines *clean eating* as emphasising the 'consumption of healthy, "pure" foods' and suggests that it 'may also reflect susceptibility to a pathological fixation with healthy eating'. In other words, clean eating includes removing any foods or food substances that are deemed to be processed or imperfect. The British Dietetic Association (BDA) even identified this trend as its number-one 'worst celeb. diet to avoid in 2017' (Ambwani et al. 2019). There's also a clear correlation between the rise of clean-eating trends and diagnosed eating disorders—something we'll discuss later as well.

**2015:** A survey of 300,000 adults in over 60 countries reports that 21 percent claimed that gluten-free living was a very important factor when choosing what to eat (Reilly 2016). In reality, only about 0.5 percent of the population medically requires a gluten-free diet (those with coeliac disease), however, many have jumped on the gluten-free bandwagon. We know many others have sensitivities or intolerances, so this isn't directed at them. But to the individuals who feel they need to be gluten free to be healthier, gluten is just a protein found in wheat—it's not toxic and doesn't lead to adverse health effects (if your body can tolerate it). Plus, a gluten-free biscuit is still a biscuit (just without gluten). In other words, gluten free isn't synonymous with *healthy*.

**2016 and beyond:** All hail the magic foods and supplements (which some may call 'superfoods'). And while *superfood* isn't a legitimate medical term, it describes certain foods with properties that are, well, super. In reality, *superfood* is a marketing term used by companies to sell their products at a higher price due to the perceived benefits—things like green tea, kale, collagen, bone broth, turmeric, and cannabidiol (CBD). Yes, each of these may have beneficial properties, but not one of them is a magic pill. Remember, no one food or nutrient, in isolation, will improve your health.

Recap:

» Many fad diets tend to be low-calorie. So while they may be successful in terms of weight loss, we know this approach isn't sustainable in the long run.

» Fad diets don't teach you anything about nutrition or how to build healthy habits. Instead, they're guided by rules, *dos* and *don'ts*. When individuals reach their goals, they often revert back to their previous habits.

» Many of these diets profit the diet's founder when individuals pay for subscriptions or buy products.

» Anything that promises quick weight loss should also come with a disclaimer that says *short-lived weight loss*.

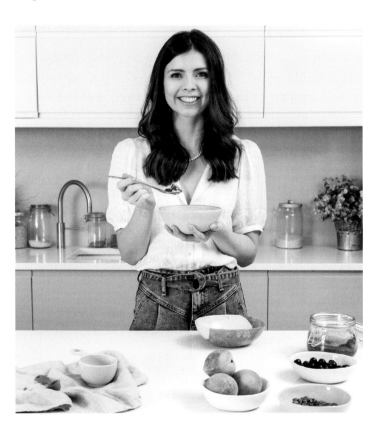

# The Price of Dieting

Let's be honest, the diet industry's goal isn't to help improve your health or lower your risk for chronic disease—it's to make money. And we mean a fork ton of money. That's why diets are unsustainable; they want you to fail. Because when you fail, you either try again or resort to another diet *(cha-ching)*.

## Can You Relate?

» **After scrolling through social media or celebrity tabloids, you look in the mirror and start to feel dissatisfied with the way you look. You may think, why don't I look like *that*?**

» **You decide you want to improve your health or lose weight, and after a quick google search or reading an ad from an influencer, you decide to start the presented diet.**

» **The diet seems a bit restrictive, so you decide to start on Monday, allowing yourself one final weekend of all the food and drinks you fear you may never have again.**

» **You buy the corresponding diet book, a monthly subscription, and branded juices, powders, and pills. You start the diet, and you feel fabulous—and look at all the weight you're losing!**

» **But then life throws you a curveball—a difficult situation. The diet didn't tell you how to prepare for this. What do you do? Do you 'cheat' on your diet? Should you just give up?**

» **You cheat on the diet because you haven't been given the tools you need to handle real-life situations and incorporate flexibility into your eating patterns. You feel guilty. You feel disappointed. You blame yourself and wonder, why don't I have enough willpower?**

» **But it's OK. You promise to start a new diet on Monday.**

Willpower isn't a real 'power' at all but rather one that was created by the diet industry to help drive profits—we'll touch on this later.

We've been exposed to diet culture for so long that we no longer trust our own abilities to make healthy decisions and improve our health on our own. We believe the only way to do this is through a labelled diet. This paradigm results in a loss of self-trust and self-compassion, a mindset that the only way to lose weight is through restriction and that our next diet will start on Monday.

But how does this affect our wallets?

According to the US Food and Drug Administration (FDA), Americans spent an estimated $30 billion a year in 1992 on diet programmes and products. In 2007 a market research firm reported that the number grew to $55 billion (Research and Markets 2019). What the actual fork?!

According to recent surveys, the average person will spend £25,000 on dieting in their lifetime (Kellow, n.d.). They should buy our book instead, ha ha!

Any guesses as to how much the diet industry is worth today?

In the US alone, the current diet industry is worth $70 forking billion (Roepe 2018). And thanks to the Global Wellness Institute and their 2017 statistics, we know that the overall global wellness economy is worth over $4.2 trillion (McGroarty 2018), with over $702 billion having been spent on healthy eating, nutrition, and weight loss (Research and Markets 2019).

Although these numbers are shockingly high and it may seem like diets are on a rise, recent research reports that the number of dieters has actually fallen in recent years thanks to the rise of the body positivity movement. Woo-hoo! But commercial diet chains and health apps are still reporting steady growth.

Quick wrap-up:

» Diets are designed to fail because the industry wants you to keep coming back for more.

» The global wellness industry was worth over $4.2 trillion as of 2017.

» The American diet industry was worth over $70 billion as of 2018.

» Although fewer individuals are turning to diets to solve their problems, the industry is still experiencing steady financial growth.

» At the end of the day, diet culture is a business—one that generates a lot of money.

# Diet Takeaway Messages

We currently live in a state of information overload, where we have the ability to find out almost anything within seconds. (Thank you, Google—or, as Bari's grandmother calls it, 'The Google'.) But with the abundance of information accessible at our fingertips, especially with regard to health and weight loss, this can often leave us feeling overwhelmed and confused. So, with the multitude of conflicting nutrition information out there, what the fork should we do?

While many current diets may be rooted in science, the quality of these studies varies (as we previously discussed). But most of the common diets do have elements of truth, which are mostly exaggerated and augmented to help sell products and false promises. And as nutrition professionals, we've seen it all. Collectively, we've worked with hundreds of clients who've spent years jumping from diet to diet, which later left them feeling confused. Should you follow a low-carb or low-fat diet? What about Whole30 and F-Factor?

To help you better understand the conflicting information out there, we created the following chart. Our aim isn't to villainise each method but to highlight what we can learn and the key points we can take away from each of these various diets. We know many of these diets have been discussed previously, but we hope you find this presentation of the research interesting.

We know this is a lot of information, but as we mentioned you in the beginning of the book, bear with us. We promise to help you see health and nutrition in a new, positive light.

| Diet | **Low-Fat**<br>(La Berge, 2008; Tobias et al. 2015; Seid and Rosenbaum 2019) |
|---|---|
| Research/ Rationale | As previously mentioned, the low-fat craze of the 90s promised improved cardiovascular health and weight loss, compared to the average diet. In theory, dietary fats, also called *lipids*, are the most energy-dense macronutrients. In other words, every gram of fat provides 9 calories (kcal), while both protein and carbohydrates provide 4 kcal/g. Thus, reducing your overall fat intake will theoretically reduce your calories consumed and result in weight loss. While there's a limited consensus on the definition of *low-fat*, it's thought that less than 30 percent kcal from fat is generally considered a low-fat diet and less than 20 percent kcal from fat is considered a very low-fat diet. |
| Pros | Various research studies do state that a low-fat diet can produce more weight loss compared to an average diet and may lower the cardiometabolic risk factors. |
| Cons | Multiple RCTs have failed to show that low-fat diets are superior to other diets. And although some studies show reducing dietary fat can result in significant weight loss compared to the average diet, *average diet* is difficult to define.<br><br>Many of the studies supporting a low-fat diet are based on self-reported measurements.<br><br>Lower triglyceride levels are used as a measure for improved cardiovascular health but may be confounded by general weight loss and not the fat intake itself, since serum triglyceride concentrations were lower in high-fat test groups.<br><br>Many low-fat food products are higher in added sugar, artificial sweeteners, and other additives. |
| Takeaway | Not all fats are created equal. While we want to reduce our overall intake of trans fat, consumption of mono- and polyunsaturated fats is linked to many positive health outcomes. Both naturally occurring saturated fat (dairy and meat) and unsaturated fat, when consumed mindfully, are part of a well-balanced diet. |

| Diet | **Low-Carb** |
|---|---|
| | (La Berge 2008; Seid and Rosenbaum 2019; Gow et al. 2014) |
| Research/ Rationale | An excess of carbohydrates causes insulin levels to rise. In the presence of high insulin levels, the body increases its fat storage capabilities. Thus, by reducing your overall carbohydrate intake, your body will reduce its fat storage and actually use excess body fat for energy. A low-carb approach is also thought to help decrease an individual's risk for type 2 diabetes mellitus (T2DM). |
| Pros | Compared to other diets, such as low-fat, a low-carb diet has been shown to report significant long-term weight loss. |
| Cons | The lack of well-controlled inpatient studies makes it hard to determine whether a low-carb approach produces any long-term significant difference compared to a low-calorie diet. |
| | At this time, current evidence doesn't suggest a low-carb (or low-fat) approach for sustained and long-term weight loss. |
| Takeaway | Being conscious of your overall sugar intake is important, especially sugars from overly processed foods. But carbohydrates aren't the enemy. Complex carbohydrates, such as lentils, legumes, potatoes, whole-grain breads, and brown rice are great sources of fibre and essential vitamins and minerals. Just remember, fruits and vegetables are also carbohydrates and packed with an abundance of important nutrients. But minimising prolonged and continuous insulin spikes from excess simple sugars can help to reduce your risk for T2DM and other chronic illnesses and help you maintain a healthy weight. |

| Diet | **Atkins** |
|---|---|
| | (Seid and Rosenbaum 2019; Atkins, n.d.; Harper, Larsen, and Astrup (2004) 2005; Gardner et al. 2007) |
| Research/ Rationale | The Akins diet, another low-carb approach, has been shown to improve insulin sensitivity and improve blood-glucose levels. |
| | According to Gardner et al. (2007), the Atkins diet was more successful at producing weight loss and favourable metabolic effects over 12 months compared to other diets. |
| Pros | Limited long-term data is available, due to Atkins's strict and unsustainable rules. |
| | A recent systematic review of low-carb diets (including Atkins) reveals that the weight loss achieved is directly associated with the duration of the diet and restriction of overall calorie intake, not the decrease of carbohydrates. |
| Cons | Limited long-term data is available, due to Atkins's strict and unsustainable rules. |
| | A recent systematic review of low-carb diets (including Atkins) reveals that the weight loss achieved is directly associated with the duration of the diet and restriction of overall calorie intake, not the decrease of carbohydrates. |

*(continued)*

*(continued)*

| | |
|---|---|
| **Takeaway** | As with the other low-carb approaches, it's undoubtedly important to be mindful of your overall simple-carbohydrate intake. Additionally, the Atkins diet and other low-carb approaches have shown us that when you decrease your carbohydrates you inadvertently increase your protein and fat, which help you feel fuller for longer. While the Atkins diet is restrictive and requires you to count carbohydrates (and leads to a detrimental fixation on—and fear of—carbohydrates), it does highlight that all dietary fat may have previously been wrongly villainised in terms of adverse health effects. But this low-carb approach appears to be restrictive and unsustainable in the long run. |

| | |
|---|---|
| **Diet** | **Keto**<br>(Goswami and Sharma 2019) |
| **Research/ Rationale** | The keto (ketogenic) diet is a high-fat and very low-carb approach, where 70–90 percent of your daily calories come from fat.<br><br>The premise of the keto diet is to put your body in a state of ketosis, which means that in the absence of glucose (carbohydrates) your body will shift to burning ketones (fat storage) for energy. |
| **Pros** | Like other low-carb approaches, the keto diet improves glycaemic control (blood sugars levels) by reducing fasted blood-glucose levels. Additionally, studies suggest the keto diet may have benefits in terms of weight loss, T2DM, Alzheimer's, and metabolic syndrome.<br><br>Moreover, the research supports the keto diet as an effective antiseizure intervention for children with epilepsy. |
| **Cons** | As with many new diets, the long-term data is lacking. But due to the keto diet's restrictive and inflexible nature, individuals on the diet have reported struggling to maintain these eating patterns over time.<br><br>The keto diet requires some social compromises, which also lends to its unsustainable nature.<br><br>Additionally, as it's a very low-carb diet, individuals following the keto diet are at higher risk for failing to meet their dietary-fibre intake. |
| **Takeaway** | Diets with strict rules are unrealistic in the long term and require many mental and physical sacrifices in terms of weight loss. For specific and short-term results, the keto diet may have its place, but the long-term results are unknown.<br><br>But the keto diet is an approved course of treatment for children with a specific type of epilepsy and should be followed only under the supervision of a registered dietitian or specialised medic. |

| | |
|---|---|
| **Diet** | **Paleo**<br><br>(Fenton and Fenton 2016; Obert et al. 2017; de Menezes et al. 2019) |
| **Research/ Rationale** | The paleo diet stems from the hypothesis that our diet should mirror the diet our ancestors ate when human evolution ceased. It's proposed that the paleo diet best supports our genetics and can decrease diseases associated with our modern lifestyle and diet.<br><br>According to the paleo diet, only foods that were present in the hunter-gatherer era should be consumed, such as meat, fruit, and vegetables. But dairy, grains, sugar, alcohol, salt, and processed foods should be eliminated. |
| **Pros** | With an emphasis on fruit, vegetables, healthy fats, and protein, the paleo diet is rich in many nutrients while eliminating processed foods. In 2019, a systematic review concluded that the paleo diet did help individuals lose weight and improve other metabolic indices in the short term. |
| **Cons** | The original research papers supporting the paleo diet have several flaws, including nonrandomised control groups and the overstatement of certain results.<br><br>Additionally, while this diet supports the consumption of many nutritious foods, the exclusion of dairy, legumes, and grains for improved health isn't justified in the research.<br><br>In order for science to support the claims made by the paleo diet, more RCTs with larger populations and durations are needed. |
| **Takeaway** | There's no doubt that a diet rich in fruit, vegetables, healthy fats, and protein has positive health benefits. And while reducing the amount of processed food in our overall diet is important, there's little to no evidence stating we need to exclude dairy, legumes, or grains (unless medically necessary). |

| | |
|---|---|
| **Diet** | **Zone**<br><br>(Cheuvront 2003; Gardner et al. 2007) |
| **Research/ Rationale** | Dr. Sears' Zone Diet is designed to place individuals in the optimal 'zone' to lose weight and reduce inflammation. This is accomplished by adhering to the Zone Diet's macronutrient breakdown of daily calories: 40 percent carbohydrates, 30 percent protein, and 30 percent fat. This ratio of protein to carbohydrates is advertised to help reduce the insulin-to-glucagon ratio, which is thought to be helpful for managing inflammation and reducing the risk of developing chronic diseases. The Zone Diet also promotes enhanced immunity, increased physical and mental performance, increased longevity, and weight loss. |
| **Pros** | The Zone Diet promotes balanced meals, especially with regard to protein and carbohydrates. As the diet insists that you should consume carbohydrates low on the glycaemic index and pair them with protein, sugars are released into the blood at a slower rate, leaving you feeling fuller for longer. |

*(continued)*

*(continued)*

| | |
|---|---|
| Cons | While the Zone Diet promotes balanced macronutrients, the literature suggests that the diet fails to back up several claims, especially with regard to inflammation and weight loss. |
| | Additionally, the Zone Diet requires an increased level of planning and counting to adequately ensure the individuals are entering the zone. This preoccupation with macronutrients may have negative mental consequences. |
| Takeaway | While 'macrocounting' may be a waste of time, the Zone Diet does promote a balanced intake of all macronutrients (protein, carbohydrates, and fat). Reaching the optimal zone, however, may require an unnecessary amount of time spent calculating the specific macronutrients. While this approach doesn't demonise certain foods, it does place a strong emphasis on microcounting your meals. But the true composition of the food promoted in this diet is balanced. |

| | |
|---|---|
| Diet | **Whole30** |
| Research/ Rationale | Whole30 is a 30-day elimination diet that involves completely giving up common 'irritants' to the body, such as alcohol, sugar, artificial sweeteners, grains, dairy, and legumes. After the 30 days, you can slowly reincorporate these foods into your routine, one at a time, which can help identify if any of them cause digestive discomfort. |
| Pros | Some individuals have reported improved digestive health, energy levels, and weight loss. |
| Cons | This diet isn't based on any scientific research and is in fact based only on anecdotal evidence. |
| | Whole30 is highly restrictive and requires individuals to cut out entire food groups, which increases the risk for nutrient deficiencies. As this diet is carried out without the supervision of a healthcare professional, many individuals prolong the elimination past 30 days and increase their risk for nutrient deficiencies. |
| | Many of the eliminated food groups have correlated with positive health outcomes in multiple research studies. |
| Takeaway | If you struggle with digestive issues, an elimination diet can be an effective course of treatment. But this should be initiated only after several other recommendations have failed to yield results and only under the supervision of a qualified health professional. |
| | But being mindful of your overall alcohol, sugar, and artificial-sweetener intake may be helpful in terms of weight loss and overall health. |

| Diet | **F-Factor** |
|---|---|
| | (F-Factor, n.d.; Simpson and Campbell 2015; Bourassa et al. 2016) |
| Research/ Rationale | The F-Factor approach was created by a registered dietitian and promotes high fibre and lean protein for weight loss. |
| | 'The F-Factor approach focuses on combining lean proteins with high-fiber carbohydrates, which are low in calories and keep you feeling full throughout the day' (F-Factor, n.d.). |
| Pros | A diet rich in fibre is undoubtedly healthy, especially because, as we previously mentioned, the average intake is around 14 g per day. (The RDA is 30 g). Adequate fibre intake has been linked to healthy weight management, improved blood glucose levels, increased immunity, decreased adverse gastrointestinal symptoms, improved heart health, and regular bowel movements. |
| | The F-Factor diet claims you won't be asked to eliminate carbs, protein, fats, or even alcohol. |
| Cons | While the F-Factor claims to not be a diet, you do have to track and log your net-carb intake (carbohydrates minus fibre equals net carbs). Also, F-Factor-approved meal swaps include swapping out spaghetti for courgette (zucchini) noodles and toast for fibre-rich crackers. While there's nothing wrong with courgette noodles or fibre biscuits, it seems that promotion of high-fibre foods decreases your food freedom. |
| | Additionally, the F-Factor website says you can 'eat carbs' and 'work out less'. This statement implies that eating carbohydrates is problematic and that exercise is a punishment. |
| | Furthermore, there have been no scientific studies comparing the health benefits of the F-Factor diet to other diets, especially low-calorie diets. |
| Takeaway | There's no doubt that fibre is important, especially because 9 out of 10 people don't meet their daily fibre needs. But it seems that the F-Factor diet uses fibre as a guise to limit your overall calories in order to lose weight: Fill up on high-fibre foods that are low in calories. It's important to remember that no nutrient should ever be put on a pedestal—it's all about balance. With that being said, fibre is extremely important and should be consumed through a wide range of plant foods (not promoted through processed biscuits or websites selling supplements). |

| Diet | **Mediterranean** |
|---|---|
| | (Mancini et al. 2016; Godos et al. 2019; Martini 2019; Galbete et al. 2018; Esposito et al. 2015) |
| Research/ Rationale | Though it's truly not a fad diet, we wanted to include the Mediterranean diet here to highlight how guidelines without restrictions or rules can be beneficial. |
| | The Mediterranean diet is characterised by the following: |
| | 1. Increased consumption of olive oil, whole-grain cereals, legumes, vegetables, and fruit. |
| | 2. Moderate consumption of wine, fish, and dairy products. |
| | 3. Decreased consumption of highly processed foods, refined grains, and sugar. |
| Pros | There's robust research to support the Mediterranean diet and its positive effects on cardiovascular disease, cognitive health, longevity, mental-health disorders, risk and management of diabetes, and other metabolic conditions. |
| | In terms of weight loss, in a 12-month follow-up study, the Mediterranean diet produced greater sustained weight loss when compared to other diets, such as a low-fat diet. Additionally, the Mediterranean diet has high adherence rates due to its lack of restriction. |
| Cons | Although the Mediterranean diet is supported in the research, for improved health outcomes, it's not exempt from its research flaws. Several studies use different scores to assess the adherence of the diet, which makes it difficult to compare. |
| | Additionally, there's inconsistency in the categorisation of food within the Mediterranean diet research. Inconsistencies can decrease the validity of the research. |
| Takeaway | The Mediterranean diet works because it focuses on what to include in your overall intake, not what you need to eliminate. This style of eating focuses on diversity and an abundance of nutritious foods without counting any specific nutrients. |

| Diet | **Intermittent Fasting** |
|---|---|
| | (Patterson et al. 2015; Rynders et al. 2019; Obert et al. 2017) |
| Research/ Rationale | Intermittent fasting (IF) may be relatively new, but it seems like everyone is trying it these days. IF involves intentionally restricting your consumption to specific times of the day or extending the time between each meal. IF comes in many different forms, whether it's restricting your intake for two to three days per week or limiting your intake to only six to eight hours per day. |
| | The strategy of IF is for individuals to consume less energy (fewer calories) during their 'feeding times' and not compensate for their energy deficit. IF also proposes that, over time, hunger levels decline. IF is thought to result in metabolic adaptations over time, such as prioritising fat metabolism (fat oxidation), which preserves lean muscle mass and sustains weight loss. |
| | Additionally, there's some research hypothesising that prolonged fasts improve the circadian rhythm and gastrointestinal microbiota. |

*(continued)*

*(continued)*

| | |
|---|---|
| Pros | Dieters are attracted to IF because, unlike many diets, they don't have to restrict calories (only the hours in a day they're allowed to eat). |
| | Rodent studies suggest that alternate-day fasts (ADFs) alleviate the results of nonrestricted high-fat feedings. In other words, ADF resulted in a lower-fat mass and lower insulin and leptin levels while improving glucose tolerance. |
| Cons | The main flaw in the IF research is the lack of well-designed RCTs in humans. Currently, a large majority of the research is based on rodent experiments. |
| | Additionally, the lack of standardised terminology with regard to IF makes generalisations difficult. Furthermore, there lacks strong evidence that intermittent energy restriction (IER) produces more weight loss and body-fat loss compared to continuous energy restriction (CER), or a low-calorie diet. |
| | Due to the restrictive nature of IF, many find this approach unsustainable. For example, a recent study rates IF with an average difficulty score of 7 out of 10 (10 being a regiment that's extremely difficult to stick to every day), and 57 percent of those reporting felt they couldn't have maintained the IF protocol beyond the 10-week intervention. |
| | Also, there's a lack of robust research to support the claims that IF improves combatting cardiovascular disease, cancer, Alzheimer's, and other chronic diseases, due insufficient long-term data. |
| Takeaway | While some individuals may be unconsciously intermittently fasting (eating their first meal around noon), the health claims around IF are just not sustained in the research (as of yet). As there's a lack of long-term human studies, we're unable to generalise the results from animal studies to humans. So if you find yourself not hungry until noon, that's great. But please don't ignore your hunger cues in the pursuit of IF. Specifically, if you have a poor relationship with food, IF may exacerbate negative behaviours or thoughts. |
| | Refer to the Minnesota Starvation Experiment case study for more interesting information. |

| | |
|---|---|
| Diet | **Alkaline** |
| | (Schwalfenberg 2012; Tobey 1936; Fenton et al. 2009; Passey 2017) |
| Research/ Rationale | The alkaline diet proposes that humans need to increase their consumption of alkaline foods and decrease their consumption of acidic foods, to improve their health and prevent disease. |
| | Alkaline foods include fruit, nuts, legumes, and vegetables, while acidic foods include meat, poultry, fish, dairy, eggs, and alcohol. |
| Pros | Diets rich in fruit, nuts, legumes, and vegetables are diverse and balanced. |
| | Additionally, there's a niche area of research showing that consuming alkaline-based foods may benefit individuals who have chronic kidney disease (CKD). But this is because the kidneys are responsible for buffering your urine and blood. Maintaining the blood's pH levels is imperative and can be affected only by your kidneys (and lungs). |

*(continued)*

*(continued)*

| | |
|---|---|
| Cons | There's no conclusive or robust evidence showing that following the alkaline diet can improve your health and reduce your risk for disease. |
| Takeaway | Consuming fruit, vegetables, legumes, and nuts is important with regard to ensuring you have a wide range of nutrients. But this doesn't mean you can't have acidic foods, such as meat, fish, dairy, and eggs. Thankfully, we're equipped with kidneys and lungs, both of which are responsible for maintaining specific pH levels in our bodies, regardless of the pH found in the food we consume. |

| | |
|---|---|
| Diet | **Juice**<br><br>(Obert et al. 2017; Esfahani et al. 2011; Sweeney et al. 1993) |
| Research/ Rationale | 'Juicing', or following a juice cleanse, consists of consuming nothing but juice from fresh fruit and vegetables. As the juice is high in antioxidants, many believe this detox is important to cleanse your body and improve your health. Many use juice cleanses to jump start their weight-loss journey. |
| Pros | Many individuals will lose weight when following a juice cleanse as they aren't consuming solid food for a prolonged period of time. |
| Cons | While a juice cleanse will result in weight loss, this is often not sustainable in the long run as it lacks sufficient nutrients (especially protein). Any weight loss is a direct result of extreme calorie deficit as juice cleanses are extremely restrictive.<br><br>Also, when you put fruit or vegetables through a juicer, you remove the pulp, which houses the fibre.<br><br>Plus there's a lack of significant evidence to support that consuming fruit juices and vegetable juices improves your overall health and decreases your risk for disease. |
| Takeaway | Ensuring you have fruits and vegetables in your diet is imperative as they provide essential vitamins and minerals and are linked to improved health outcomes. But you don't need to have fruit and vegetable juices to improve your health. Consuming a whole fruit or a vegetable, such as an apple or a leafy salad, provides more nutritional impact.<br><br>Additionally, no food or food substance has the ability to detox or cleanse your body. Thankfully, we have a liver and kidneys to do that for us. |

# The Bigger Picture

While there are numerous diets out there, all with various rules, there are some key themes in this chart. The majority of diets argue for good quality protein, plenty of vegetables, and some form of carbohydrates (fibre). The rest of the plate (or day) is truly what varies. Most diets argue for a decreased intake of processed foods, sugar, and alcohol. But, as you've read, most diets are unsustainable in the long run, specifically because the rules are too strict.

The common theme of protein, vegetables, and whole grains in these diets is important. These foods help provide some of the essential nutrients we need. Plus, they help keep our blood-sugar levels stable, which is important for lowering our risk of disease. But these aren't the only nutrients we should be consuming. Don't forget that while food provides us with fuel it's also something to enjoy. Food provides pleasure and enjoyment, which is an integral part of a healthy lifestyle.

So what the fork should we do?

Well, we're about to break it down for you really simply.

Overall, your intake should consist of high-quality protein, healthy fats, and whole-grain carbohydrates with plenty of fruit and vegetables. There's no counting (macros or calories) involved, and there are definitely no restrictions. We can't deny that some foods have more nutrients than others (avocado vs. chocolate cake), but that doesn't mean one is better than the other. They're simply different. Of course we want to prioritise the nutrient-dense foods because they help our bodies thrive and provide us with the necessary nutrients, but that doesn't mean the other foods have to be villainised or cut out.

## What the fork is a high-quality protein?

A high-quality protein is one that provides all the essential amino acids and has those amino acids available to us through digestion. This is key when it comes to ensuring our body functions properly. Not every protein you enjoy has to be 'high-quality', but it's important to ensure you're having enough of these proteins to prevent any deficiencies. Here are some high-quality proteins:

» **meat (including poultry)**
» **fish**
» **eggs**
» **quinoa**
» **soya**

To be honest, when it comes to what you should eat, the bigger picture is all about flexibility without guilt or shame. It's about listening to your body, whether it's telling you to have veggie stir-fry or a vanilla milkshake. It's about not compensating via restriction or exercise for enjoying foods that are less nutrient dense. We'll talk a lot more about this in future chapters, so stay tuned.

But for now, just remember that the majority of the diets listed in the chart (apart from the Mediterranean diet) require you to cut out (eliminate) foods. Such restriction is inevitably unsustainable. Moreover, many of the perceived benefits from following these diets aren't even substantiated in the research.

So ditch the diets and ditch the rules. Focus on balance, diversity, and flexibility.

# Personalised Nutrition

Before you dive right into the next chapter (another good one!), we want to talk about personalised nutrition. It's important to remember that we're all unique and what works for one person may not work for another. In other words, we each have a unique set of DNA with different genetic factors. This will affect our personal preferences, how we break down and store nutrients, and so much more. Accounting for these unique differences is what makes public nutrition recommendations so difficult.

Even identical twins, who share the same DNA and genetic factors, can respond differently to specific eating styles due to epigenetics. Epigenetics describes the environmental impact on genes, which can turn the genes on or off or even alter gene expression. So, while identical twins have the same DNA, their genes can be expressed differently. This accounts for differences in twins' individual risks for developing type 2 diabetes, cancer, and even autism (Castillo-Fernandez, Spector, and Bell 2014).

We specifically want to point this out because even two people with the same DNA can have severely different outcomes; it's important to not compare yourself to the others around you. Just because your friend Nicole feels great on a low-carb diet doesn't mean you should be jumping to ditch bread.

Quick wrap-up:

» There are several conflicting diets out there that each claim to be the best with regard to weight management, improving overall health, and minimising risk of disease.

» Many of these diets and their claims are unsubstantiated in the research, specifically due to difficulty in adherence to the strict rules.

» Most diets focus on protein, vegetables, and fibre, which remain important and integral to a healthy lifestyle.

» It's important to prioritise nutrient-dense foods but not at the risk of cutting out less-nutrient-dense foods.

» Healthy eating patterns include balance, diversity, and flexibility without rules or restrictions.

» We're all unique and shouldn't compare our eating habits to others'.

# Finding Balance

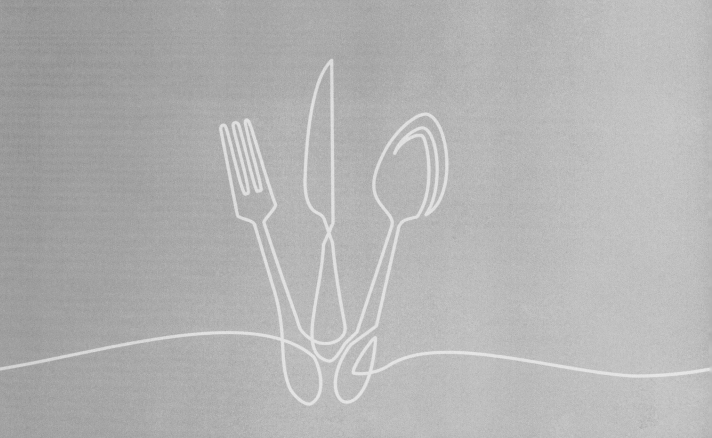

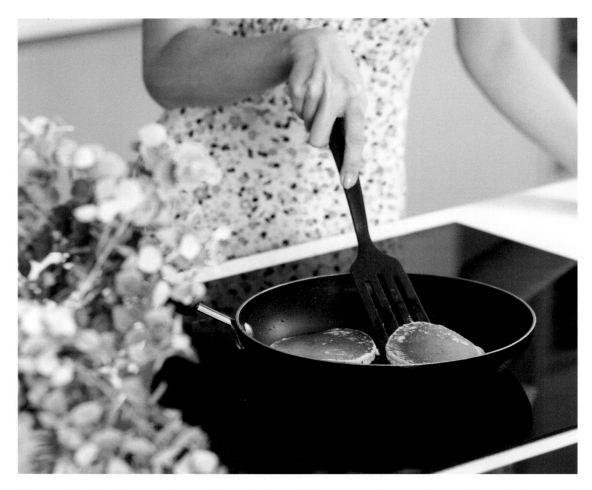

The word *healthy* often gets dragged through the mud, thus, most of us now have no idea what it actually means. For example, maple syrup was once named the healthier version of sugar. Sorry, guys, but sugar is sugar, and your body can't tell the difference between granulated sugar and a syrup form of sugar—they get metabolised in the same way. You should just choose what you prefer the taste of. Often in the pursuit of 'health', we forget about actual health—we might be guilty of at some point focusing on what we look like as opposed to how we feel, and neglecting mental health definitely isn't what well-being is about. So let's break down what health actually encompasses and how you can determine what health looks like for you. This can help you enjoy food whilst making informed choices with regard to the best way you can support your own well-being (physically and mentally).

**Diet culture** is basically a collection of beliefs that have been solidified by environmental messages telling us that weight loss equals health and that being thin should be a priority.

# How to Find the Balance Between Eating for Health as Well as Enjoyment

A well-balanced diet is important for good health, but what do we mean when we say *balance*? The word is often thrown around, particularly on social media, however, our lives are so busy and we're all so unique that balance can't possibly mean the same for each individual. Nevertheless, when it comes to food, it's possible to do what works for you and find the version of balance that makes you feel good about yourself. We're here to give you some guidance with regard to eating for health and enjoyment and to let you know that all your choices (and preferences) are valid. Each food group serves a different purpose for the body, whether it be physically or mentally. For example, carbohydrates supply our brains and our bodies with energy. But food isn't just energy—it's enjoyment. You can choose foods from different food groups because you enjoy them and they taste good. We've both worked with clients who'd forgotten that food can actually be enjoyable, because a lot of people are so focused on a weight-loss goal. We want to educate you and help you fall in love with food at the same time. This way, it'll be easier for you to identify what your definition of *balance* is.

We have an 'all food is fit' outlook on food. This means that an overall diet should be rich in all the nutrients we explained in the 'Nutrition Basics' chapter, having plenty of fibre, omega-3s and high-quality protein but not putting any food off-limits, meaning you can and should enjoy foods that are perhaps less nutrient dense too. Balance includes everything from delicious veggie-packed buddha bowls and overnight oats to smoothies, lentils, and avocados but also includes chocolate, G and Ts, fries, and brownies. Balance within the diet is key to an overall healthy relationship with food as it encourages individuals to not look at food in such black-and-white terms and to avoid restriction of a certain food or food group.

To find your healthy balance, try and put on the back burner any weight-loss goal you might have. When you don't feel like you're on a diet, you give yourself the opportunity to identify what foods you like and what foods make you feel good. A lot of people are usually concerned that they may want only 'unhealthy' foods. But that's not how the body works. When you truly listen to your body, you'll likely be pleasantly surprised to find that you enjoy a variety of foods. Be prepared that this might take some time. If you're someone who's spent years dieting, you may enter a period where you find you eat more than you need—this is your body's response to restriction. But once you legalise all foods (read Ten Principles of IE in the 'What About Intuitive Eating?' section), the foods you once restricted will likely lose their appeal and you'll feel confident in knowing that when your body feels like eating a certain food you can enjoy it without feeling the need to binge on it. Once you've spent some time deciding what foods you love and what makes you feel energised physically and mentally, you can start to incorporate your nutrition knowledge (that we hope you'll have obtained from this book). Yes, it's so important for your overall well-being that you don't deprive yourself of foods, but we also know it's important to make sure you're getting adequate amounts of a variety of nutrients. You don't have to eat in a super-strict way to call yourself healthy. Half our problem is feeling judged and comparing ourselves to other people. But nutrition isn't black-and-white. There's a grey area that you can feel your best at, and that grey area will look very different for another individual. We're all unique, so focus on you and your body and fork what other people are doing.

## FINDING BALANCE IN LIFE

How do we find balance in life? That's the million dollar question. Although we're nutrition professionals, we've had some experience with regard to feeling overwhelmed in life and like we're either pushing ourselves too much or not enough. Bari has a full-time job as well as running her Instagram, @barithedietitian, and Sophie runs her own business (Sophie's Healthy Kitchen) and runs @sophieshealthykitchen. Keeping up with work, networking, seeing friends, spending time with family, being full-time dog mums—we too struggle to find balance. Aside from diet, we need to consider stress levels, sleep, movement, and just feeling like our best selves.

These lifestyle factors are all covered in the next chapter, but we have some personal tips of our own that may help, too.

### Top Tips

» Make lists. **Lists are so damn helpful when you're trying to work through the 'mess' in your brain. Write one out on a Monday morning, write out your shopping list, write out what life admin stuff you need to do. There's nothing more satisfying than crossing off things on a to-do list. (We think so anyway!)**

» Make time for yourself. **Some people are scared to stop, 'losing' time that could have been spent being productive. But think of it this way—when you put aside 20–30 minutes to have your coffee, have a bath, or go for a walk, you feel much more focused and productive when you come back to what you were doing. Sometimes it might require a whole day or even a week to 'reset' yourself, but make sure you're not pushing yourself to the point of exhaustion.**

» Set goals. **Whether they're short- or long-term goals, it can be really motivating to work towards something specific, and there doesn't always have to be a timeline attached to it. A goal could be as small as making sure you get out for a walk every day or as big as wanting to write your own book one day. They say if you believe something, you're halfway there. (Not too sure who 'they' are, but we've heard good things.)**

# Black-and-White Thinking Surrounding Food

So how the fork do we eat for our well-being as well as not obsess over the foods that are 'good' for us and enjoy eating at the same time? Diet culture has made that seem pretty impossible, huh? Yes, there's research behind certain foods and certain ways of eating, but the problem is that we're often hit with the headlines, and unless you're a researcher or health professional, you don't tend to read the journal articles they came from. For example, 'Omega-3s Can Reduce Your Risk of Alzheimer's'—now, there's a substantial amount of research suggesting this may be true, however, this isn't to say that just by adding sources of omega-3s to your diet you won't suffer from Alzheimer's later in life, because there are other elements to brain health, such as antioxidant intake, levels of stress and anxiety, and exercise. We often take away a little bit of information and forget about the overall picture—the one that makes up well-being.

A piece of cake isn't going to make you put on weight, and it certainly doesn't make you unhealthy. A salad isn't going to make you lose weight and doesn't make you healthy. We need to stop labelling foods as such and stop separating them into different categories. Let's look at it this way: A piece of cake is pretty damn tasty and can also be very satisfying. It's nice to enjoy a piece of cake when you feel like it, because it makes you feel good. A salad can be really delicious. On a summer's day, a nice fresh salad with some lentils and a variety of veg makes for a nutrient-dense meal. This can make you feel good too. See what we did there? Food is enjoyable and satisfying. The moment you start categorising these foods, it takes that enjoyment away from eating, because the likelihood is that you're not eating it because you want to; you're eating it because you think you should. Being in a diet mentality can encourage an all-or-nothing approach to food. One study found that those who were prone to black-and-white thinking about food were more likely to restrict their food intake in order to try and control their weight (Palascha et al. 2015).

If you're reading this book, you're likely looking for answers because restriction, food rules, and black-and-white thinking about food hasn't been working for you. We feel you. Know that you're not alone and we've all been there. It might seem scary, ditching the rules and actually trusting your body, but once you push past the initial fear, it's so worth it.

## CHALLENGING THE FOOD RULES

We've likely all had 'food rules' at some point in our lives. You might still have them. They've been created over time, maybe to comfort you, make you feel more in control of your body, or help you achieve a weight-loss goal. But can you honestly say that food rules contribute to a happy, healthy, and well-balanced life? Getting rid of food rules is an important step if you want a healthy relationship with food. (We explain this more in our 'What About Intuitive Eating?' section.)

## Top Tips

» **Identify Negative Thoughts**

Before you start to challenge your food rules, you need to actually identify them first. They might be so constant that you may not realise how ingrained they are. So be mindful of your thoughts about food and your decision making. You might find it useful to write these down.

» **Change the Wording**

Once you've identified any irrational beliefs or words regarding food (words like should, can't, and must), you can start to reword them. For example, instead of thinking, I shouldn't be hungry two hours after breakfast, try: Maybe I didn't eat enough at breakfast. I'll honour my hunger and satisfy my body. You need to start talking to yourself in a more positive way and learn to trust that your body is capable of sending the right signals.

» **Implement the Change**

Keep on top of these thoughts. No matter how many times you need to fight them, keep at it. They'll become less significant over time.

Have you ever been doing your food shop, walking down the aisles, with a voice in your head telling you to check calories, compare foods, and pick the 'healthier' or low-fat option? Or do you ever feel a little peckish in between meals and hear that voice say, 'Don't be greedy'? That's the food police—a term used in the non-diet world that refers to unreasonable rules in your head. But you want to be healthier, right? So why not listen to those voices? We'll tell you why: those voices have been formed off the back of diet culture, mixed messages, and confusing information. And you think that voice is trying to protect you, but it's not. It's likely causing disordered eating patterns and an unhealthy relationship with food. So how do we challenge and get rid of these unwanted thoughts that are making every decision about food miserable? Tell them to fork off! Easier said than done, but if you start to and continue to fight back, that voice will get quieter and quieter. But how do you challenge them? We've come up with some steps that we hope you'll find helpful.

# Orthorexia: When 'Healthy' Becomes Unhealthy

We both feel strongly that this topic is an important one to cover. When the idea of healthy is taken to the extreme, it really can have devastating effects, and we believe it's necessary to highlight this.

When we start to obsess over being healthy, there's a risk of the obsession developing into some form of an eating disorder (ED). Although this is not officially recognised by the *Diagnostic Statistical Manual of Mental Disorders (DSM-5)*, medical professionals are becoming more aware of what's known as orthorexia.

The term *orthorexia* was coined in 1998 and may differ from other EDs in the sense that orthorexia has less of a focus on losing weight. The research that's been done in this area suggests that individuals suffering with this type of ED are more fixated on the type of food they're eating. For example, someone with orthorexia might only eat foods that are considered 'pure' and contain an abundance of nutrients. But as a result, weight loss is likely to occur (Koven and Abry 2015).

Adopting what's perceived as such a 'clean' way of eating, will likely put you at risk of malnutrition as a result of nutrient deficiencies. It may sound healthy, but restricting your food intake based on what you believe to be clean can lead to ill health. For example, take plant-based milks—some nut milk simply contains the nut, salt, and water; therefore, the label looks less overwhelming. The labels of fortified milks contain stabilisers too. You may think these ingredients aren't pure when in fact they're safe to consume and support the nutrients added to the milk. We're not saying there's anything wrong with any type of plant-based milk, but if you're vegan, you'll likely benefit from drinking fortified milks (which usually contain calcium, vitamin B12, and magnesium).

Although the cause of orthorexia isn't clear, some studies suggest there are some risk factors. These include obsessive-compulsive disorder, a history of an ED (e.g. anorexia or bulimia), tendencies towards being a perfectionist, or any combination of the three (Varga et al. 2013; Koven and Abry 2015). If you think you may be suffering with orthorexia, please seek professional help from a registered nutritionist or dietitian and from a psychologist.

## THE ORTO-15

The ORTO-15 is a tool in the form of a questionnaire (Donini et al. 2005, e 30), to help individuals identify whether or not they may be suffering with orthorexia. Although this test has its limitations, it may work as a general assessment with regard to potentially problematic attitudes towards food. If you decide to complete the questionnaire, it might be a good idea to ignore the scoring section of the quiz as a good goal is to highlight potentially negative thought patterns only, but not to encourage self-diagnosis. Remember, you should always see your general practitioner (GP) and not rely on a quiz if you feel you may identify with any of these statements. The questionnaire is available from researchgate.net and searching for 'Orthorexia nervosa: Validation of a diagnosis questionnaire' (Dunn and Bratman 2016).

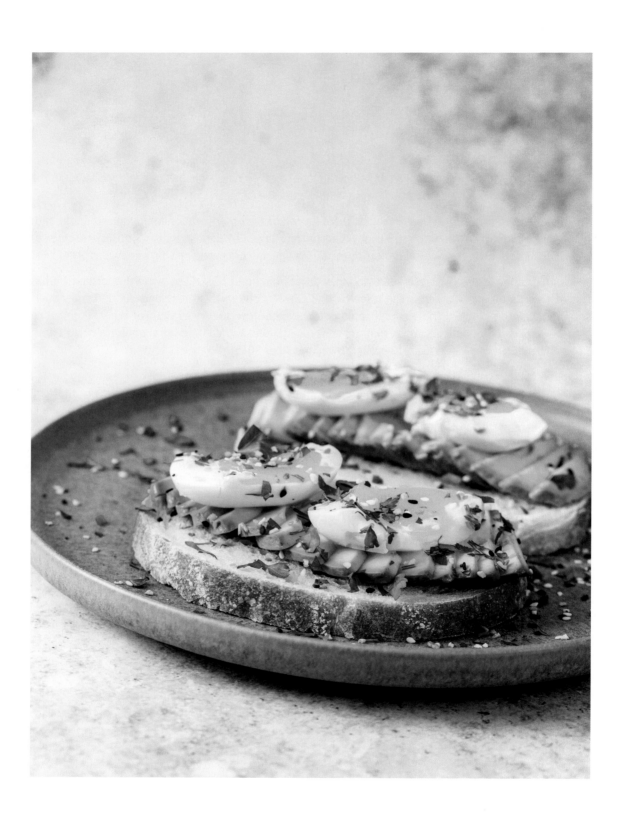

# Lifestyle Factors

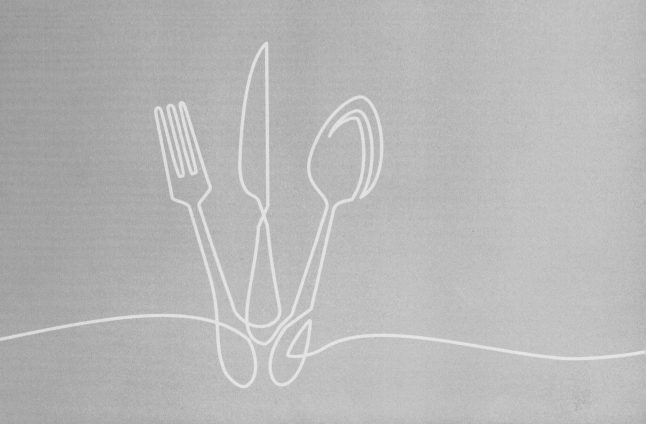

When we think about *health*, a lot of us automatically think that refers to what we eat. And whilst it's true that diet plays a huge role in well-being, there are many other factors to consider too. In this chapter, we're going to dig into the bigger picture and help you think about how you can use a number of tools to move forward in a positive way whilst enhancing your overall well-being.

# Exercise

Now, we're not sure what comes to your mind when we say *discuss exercise*, but we tend to find that people either exercise for weight loss or move to feel great. It could be both, but ideally what we want you to take away from this section is that exercise has so much more to offer than just physical benefits.

Diet culture will tell you that exercise burns fat and helps compensate for 'bad' foods you think you have or will eat that day and will perhaps even go as far as referring to sweat as the fat on your body 'crying'. Damn, what an unenjoyable way to think about a workout. We have a *Forking Wellness* podcast episode where we discuss exercise and often refer to it as *movement*. Sometimes people associate exercise with an intense workout, but you don't have to leave the gym sweating (or feeling like you're going to pass out) to say you've had a good workout. In fact, you don't even need the gym at all, because there are endless ways you can move your body to feel the benefits. Don't like the gym? Try a dance class or just dance for fun, do Pilates or yoga, swim, box, play tennis, walk your dog. Switch it up so you don't get bored and so you remember why you're moving.

Here are some evidence-based reasons to get up and move.

## MOVEMENT CAN IMPROVE YOUR MOOD

Regular exercise can change how the brain regulates feelings of stress and anxiety. Studies have shown exercise can heighten sensitivity in the brain, affecting the hormone serotonin, which can help relieve symptoms of depression. Research also indicates that when we move our bodies, chemicals known as endorphins are released, which results in a 'happy feeling' (Anderson and Shivakumar 2013). Even just going for a walk in the fresh air can help clear your mind, as studies suggest that the intensity of the workout isn't always significant. You can help improve your mood just by moving in ways you enjoy that don't seem like a chore (Meyer et al. 2016).

## MOVEMENT HELPS TO MAINTAIN HEALTHY MUSCLES AND BONES

When it comes to strengthening your muscles and bones and maintaining that strength, exercise is key. Weight-bearing exercise in particular can aid muscle building, but it's important to make sure you're eating adequate amounts of protein too. As we get older, our muscle mass and bone density, unfortunately, weaken (Boskey and Coleman 2010). Incorporating strength training into your routine can help protect your body and maintain your muscle mass (Tipton and Wolfe 2001). Additionally, strength training can reduce the risk of osteoporosis (Zulfarina et al. 2016).

## MOVEMENT MAY REDUCE THE RISK OF CHRONIC ILLNESS

Not only might exercise reduce your risk of chronic illness, but inactivity has been found to significantly increase the risk of chronic illness (Booth, Roberts, and Laye 2012). Plus, some research also shows that regular movement may help to improve cardiovascular health and insulin sensitivity and reduce high blood pressure and risk of type 2 diabetes (Slentz, Houmard, and Kraus 2009; Duscha et al. 2005; Halbert et al. 1997).

## MOVEMENT MAY HELP IMPROVE COGNITIVE FUNCTION

Exercising can help improve the function of the brain and even protect your ability to think and memorise information. Moving your body promotes blood flow to the brain and stimulates the production of brain cells (Cotman, Berchtold, and Christie 2007). It can also help maintain the structure of the brain as that may decline with age (Kirk-Sanchez and McGough 2014). Some studies even demonstrate that exercise can decrease changes in the brain, which can lead to neurodegenerative diseases, such as Alzheimer's disease (Pedrinolla, Schena, and Venturelli 2017).

## MOVEMENT MAY ENHANCE QUALITY OF SLEEP

Hopefully after reading our section on sleep (page 62), you'll understand what an important role it plays with regard to your overall well-being and that anything you can do to improve the quality of your sleep is worth doing. Moving your body regularly can actually help aid relaxation, thus preparing it for a more restful night's sleep (Kredlow et al. 2015; Driver and Taylor 2000).

Usually when we exercise, our body temperature increases. Before we fall asleep, our temperature is supposed to drop, and exercise can help regulate this process (Gilbert et al. 2004). One study in particular concludes that around 150 minutes of exercise a week can improve quality of sleep by up to 65 percent (Loprinzi and Cardinal 2011). There's no single exercise that's superior to others. Rather, it's the variety of exercise, from aerobic to resistance training, that results in improved sleep (Bonardi et al. 2016).

## MOVEMENT IMPROVES ENERGY LEVELS

Adding daily movement into our routines can really help increase our energy levels. This applies to healthy individuals as well as those suffering from chronic fatigue and even progressive illnesses (Puetz 2006; Larun et al. 2016; Payne, Wiffen, and Martin 2012).

However you choose to move, enjoyment is key. It's unlikely you'll be able to reap the benefits we've listed if you're 'dragging' yourself to the gym every day. You don't have to sweat every day, and you don't have to see exercise as a chore. We're extremely confident you can find a way to move your body that makes you feel good—you just have to explore a little and be patient with yourself. Oh, and don't compare your physical activity to someone else's.

# Stress

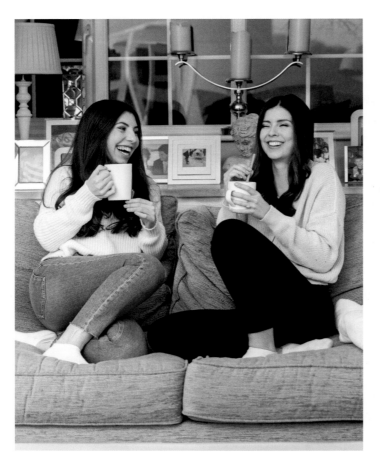

Stress is something we all experience, and there may be times in life where you feel the effects of stress on a more severe level. Stress can present itself in many different ways, whether that be physically or emotionally. In triggering situations, hormones are released that increase the rate of our breathing, sometimes making our hearts race or feel tense. This is basically our bodies making us aware of a serious or distressing situation. In that case, stress is actually a healthy and normal response. But if our stress levels stay elevated for a prolonged period of time, it may take a toll on our well-being. Severe or chronic stress may result in feelings of frustration, irritability, anxiousness, low mood or sleep disturbances (NHS 2020).

As well as affecting mental well-being, stress can play a role in disrupting the digestive system. When your body feels stressed, the increased hormone release that causes your heart rate to increase may affect the way in which you digest food, causing symptoms such as heartburn as a result of excess stomach acid. Your reaction to stress could also result in diarrhoea or constipation.

The hormone released in response to stress is known as cortisol. If cortisol levels stay elevated, it may lead to weight gain, high blood pressure, lack of energy, low mood, and even a weakened immune system (Vicennati et al. 2009; Pistollato et al. 2016; Powell et al. 2013; Buford and Willoughby 2008).

Stress can present itself in many different ways, and we all deal with it differently. It may cause physical pain, such as headaches or chest pain; it may affect your ability to focus; and it's also common to under- or overeat in times of stress. Being that stress requires a hormonal response, it may also disrupt the menstrual cycle, causing women to have delayed or even absent periods (Nagma et al. 2015).

## Top Tips to Help Manage and Reduce Stress

» **Identify Stress and What Triggers It**

Try and observe what situations trigger a stressful reaction. They could be things that happen at work, home, or in social situations. Once you've identified them, you can learn how to deal with them (Turan et al. 2015).

» **Prioritise Sleep**

The amount of and the quality of your sleep can actually influence cortisol (Hirotsu, Tufik, and Andersen 2015). Ideally, you want to establish a regular sleeping pattern and not make a habit out of napping during the day due to sleep deprivation. (Also refer to page 62.)

» **Get Up and Move to Make Yourself Feel Good**

Exercise releases feel-good endorphins and may help distract you from life's stressful situations (Mayo 2018). Make sure you choose an activity you enjoy. This could be as simple as a dog walk or as adventurous as a dance class—as long as you're enjoying it and it helps you personally to relieve stress, you're good. Yoga has also been suggested to aid in managing stress levels (Riley and Park 2015).

» **Relax**

Relaxation techniques, such as mindfulness, have been suggested to have a very positive effect when it comes to reducing cortisol levels (Matousek, Dobkin, and Pruessner 2010). Some studies have suggested that relaxing music might help (Uedo et al. 2004) along with massage therapy (Field et al. 2005). Try and figure out what helps you feel relaxed and prioritise it in times of stress.

» **Find Your Support System**

Friends and family can play a huge role in overall well-being. Make sure you're spending time with loved ones who make you feel happy (Kirschbaum et al. 1995). Happiness may also reduce cortisol (Steptoe et al. 2009).

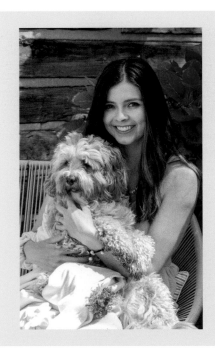

» Play With a Pet

**Interestingly, there have been numerous studies that show that having a relationship with a pet may help reduce cortisol levels. One study even goes as far as showing that some individuals felt better supported by their pet than by a human (Polheber and Matchock 2014).**

» Eat Well-Balanced Meals

**In times of stress you may be prone to 'stress eating' and tend to opt for high-sugar foods. Although there's nothing wrong with stress eating (we all do this from time to time), it'll unlikely make you feel better in the long run. Try and make sure you're including in your diet a variety of foods that will nourish your mind and body in times of stress.**

# Sleep

## WHY IS IT IMPORTANT?

Believe it or not, sleeping well is imperative to our well-being. Extensive research suggests that sleep can affect our energy levels, concentration, mood, immune system, and risk of certain diseases—all things that help determine overall health. So let's take a look at the research.

Getting a good night's sleep may impact your concentration and productivity levels. Have you ever been sitting at your desk at work finding it almost impossible to focus on anything? That may be due to lack of rest. A variety of research identifies a link between sleep and brain function. This includes your ability to perform, concentrate, and be productive (Ellenbogen 2005).

Furthermore, did you know a lack of sleep can have an effect on our physical performance? A specific study looked at over 2800 women and found that poor-quality sleep was linked to a number of factors with regard to performance: 'Objectively measured, poorer sleep was associated with worse physical function' (Goldman et al. 2007).

Some research has suggested that lack of sleep may lead to weight gain (Patel and Hu 2008). But this may be due to a number of factors. It's not as simple as equating a lack of sleep with weight gain. It's believed that sleep deprivation may influence our hormones, our motivation to exercise, or both (Di Milia, Vandelanotte, and Duncan 2013). For example, some studies have demonstrated that sleep deprivation may disrupt the hormones that regulate appetite. This refers to the hormone ghrelin, which signals the body when hungry, and leptin, the 'satiety hormone'. Some studies have indicated that lack of sleep may leave us feeling hungrier the next day, thus increasing calorie intake. It's important to note that consistent behaviours are what determine our overall well-being—a bad night's sleep doesn't mean you'll put on weight. It's what we do consistently over time that has an impact.

## HOW DIET MAY IMPACT SLEEP

Diet may determine our quality of sleep. For example, if you eat a heavy meal close to when you put your head on the pillow, your body is likely going to still be digesting food, thus making you feel uncomfortable and not ready to fall asleep. On the flip side, if you haven't eaten enough, you don't want to go to bed with a rumbling stomach. There are certain nutrients that have been associated with aiding good sleep.

**Magnesium:** Studies have found that magnesium helps activate the parasympathetic nervous system, which is what aids relaxation in the body (Wienecke and Nolden 2016). As well as sending signals to the nervous system and the brain, magnesium plays a role in regulating melatonin, the hormone that regulates the sleep cycle (Durlach et al. 2002).

If you eat an overall-balanced diet, it's likely you're getting enough of the nutrients that help aid sleep.

Magnesium is present in a variety of foods, including almonds, yoghurt, salmon, and dark chocolate

**Tryptophan:** The amino acid tryptophan can be found in protein-containing foods, and it's used by the body to help make melatonin and serotonin, the hormones that help regulate sleep (Berger, Gray, and Roth 2009). Research has indicated that a diet rich in serotonin can help improve sleep, due to increased production of melatonin. Carbohydrates like bread, potato, and rice help to stimulate the release of insulin, which clears other amino acids from the bloodstream, and this may facilitate the entry of enough tryptophan into the brain to make the necessary serotonin and melatonin (Lindseth and Murray 2016). Tryptophan can be found in poultry, fish, eggs, cheese, nuts, seeds, and milk.

Anything that's high in caffeine, sugar, or alcohol may hinder sleep.

**Omega-3:** Some studies have found that foods rich in omega-3s may help you achieve a deeper sleep (Montgomery et al. 2014). Oily fish such as salmon and mackerel are good sources of omega-3s, but omega-3s can also be found in plant sources such as walnuts, chia seeds, and flaxseeds.

## WHAT WE MEAN BY A GOOD NIGHT'S SLEEP

The research available to us suggests that anything between seven and nine hours of uninterrupted sleep is optimal, however, it's important to point out that some people are capable of needing more or less than this, but this is a general statistic that may be beneficial for most people (Lichtenstein 2015). So what counts as a good night's sleep? The National Sleep Foundation (n.d.) advises that (ideally) individuals fall asleep around 15–20 minutes after they put their heads on the pillow and that there shouldn't be long periods of the night where one is lying wide awake. A good night's sleep will usually leave you feeling refreshed in the morning and ready to start your day. You may notice you feel less alert, less productive, and perhaps more hungry (like you need more energy) if you've had a restless night.

### Top Tips for a Good Night's Sleep

» **Make sure you're in a comfortable environment.**

» **Minimise noise and turn off the TV and any lights that might come from your phone or laptop.**

» **Have a routine—try and keep the times you go to sleep and wake up similar each day.**

» **Limit your caffeine intake.**

# Hydration

A lot of people simply don't drink enough water, and from personal experience, we also see many clients who aren't staying hydrated. We believe that many underestimate the power of keeping themselves hydrated. We've all been told to drink six to eight glasses of water a day—we don't know about you, but we find this rather unhelpful—how big is the glass supposed to be? Additionally, some individuals need more or less than this amount, depending on factors such as weight, height, and physical activity levels. The Mayo Clinic states that the National Academies of Sciences, Engineering, and Medicine determined that an adequate daily fluid intake is the following:

About 15 ½ cups (3.7 L) of fluids for men

About 11 ½ cups (2.7 L) of fluids for women

This is inclusive of water, herbal teas, and food. (Coffee and sugary drinks don't count.) Your urine is a good indicator with regard to whether or not you're hydrated. Dark yellow suggests you're not drinking enough. Ideally, you want to see a very light-yellow colour when you look at your urine.

*Top Tip*

**If you're not keen on water, try adding some fresh fruit for flavour or try having herbal teas (Mayo 2017).**

How much water you need can depend on several factors, as listed in the following table.

| | |
|---|---|
| Exercise | If you're physically active and tend to break a sweat most days, you'll need to drink extra water. When working out, you should hydrate before, during, and after. (Athletes may need specific sports drinks to replenish loss of electrolytes.) |
| Environment | If you live in a hot climate or are on holiday where you'll likely sweat more than you're used to, you'll need to compensate. |
| Current Health | When ill, our bodies lose fluids (usually through vomiting, diarrhoea, or excessive sweating), meaning you'll need to take special care with regard to keeping the body hydrated. Some GPs may even recommend an oral drink to help. Other conditions, such as urinary tract infections, may also require you to drink more water. |
| Pregnant or Breastfeeding | It's important for pregnant women (and those breastfeeding) to stay well hydrated. Always consult your GP to make sure you're looking after yourself. |

## WHY HYDRATION MATTERS

Hydration matters for the following reasons:

» Your body is approximately 60 percent water. Your body and brain can be largely influenced with regard to how hydrated you are (Popkin, D'Anci, and Rosenberg 2010).

» Studies demonstrate that physical performance may be seriously affected if you allow your body's water content to drop by just 2 percent (Murray 2007).

» Research shows that even mild dehydration can influence the function of your brain in a negative way, which includes feelings of anxiety, fatigue, and poor-working memory and may also result in headaches (Pross et al. 2013; Cian et al. 2001).

» Constipation is something most of us will suffer from at some point in life, but if you're someone who struggles with regular bowel movements, it may be wise to ensure you're drinking enough water as not staying hydrated may be affecting it (Murakami et al. 2007).

# How Food Can Affect Mood

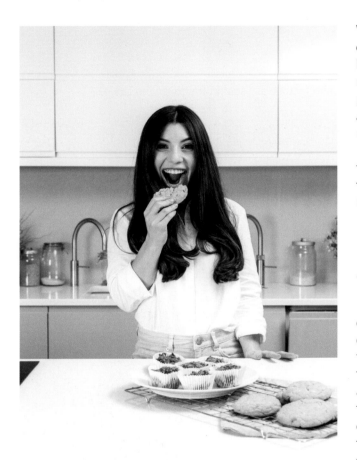

What we eat can have a significant impact on how we feel. Food not only fuels the body but also plays an essential role with regard to fuelling the brain, too. Making positive changes to your diet may enhance and regulate your mood, provide you with more energy, and help you concentrate. Lack of nutrients in the diet can lead to fatigue and poor brain function. So let's talk about what nutrients are needed to help make sure you feel good mentally.

## CARBS

It's thought that the brain uses 20 percent of all energy needed by the body. The glucose from carbohydrate-containing foods provides adequate fuel for the brain to function properly. If you've ever tried a low-carb diet and felt like you couldn't think straight, now you know why. Lack of glucose in the blood will result in tiredness, weakness, and low mood. Good sources include breads, whole grains, starchy vegetables, and fruit.

## B VITAMINS

Whilst there's no single food that can cure depression, B vitamins have been strongly linked to fighting symptoms of depression and anxiety (Lewis et al. 2013). There's also evidence to suggest that B vitamins may enhance a person's response to treatment alongside antidepressants (Almeida et al. 2014). Whole grains, meats, eggs, dairy products, and plant foods such as legumes, nuts, and leafy greens all provide B vitamins, so try and get as much variety as possible.

## TRYPTOPHAN

Tryptophan is an amino acid that's necessary to help make serotonin. Serotonin is a neurotransmitter that helps regulate mood and is also important for sleep, emotion, and appetite regulation. Foods that contain tryptophan include salmon, poultry, eggs, tofu, nuts, and seeds (Jenkins et al. 2016).

## OMEGA-3

There is a lot of research linking omega-3 intake to reduced symptoms of depression and also reduced risk of neurodegenerative diseases, such as Alzheimer's. Omega-3s are an essential part of the diet, so if you don't consume foods rich in omega-3s often, it may be worth supplementing. Foods that contain omega-3 include oily fish, such as salmon and mackerel, walnuts, flaxseed, and eggs enriched with omega-3s (O' Donovan et al. 2019; Larrieu and Layé 2018).

## $H_2O$

Water is essential to helping our bodies function properly, and when it comes to our mood, dehydration can have a negative effect. Not drinking enough water throughout the day can lead to headaches, low mood, poor concentration, and irritability. (See more on page 64.)

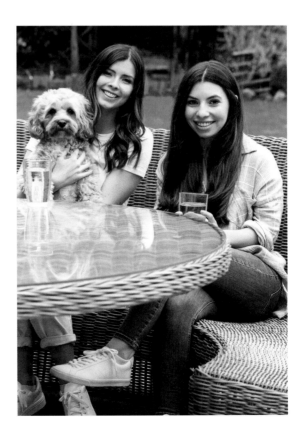

If you're eating a variety of carbohydrates (mostly whole grains), proteins, and nutrients from diverse fruits, veg, and other plant foods, you're likely to be supporting your body's needs. Eating regularly may also help to keep energy levels stable throughout the day (Arens 2020).

# What About Caffeine?

Caffeine is an extremely popular, widely consumed stimulant, and people choose to include it in their day-to-day life for many different reasons. But how might it affect your mood? This largely depends on your caffeine tolerance. Some people have a coffee and feel great. Some feel great and then experience a sudden drop in energy, which begs the question, Is it worth it? Some individuals have a very low tolerance for caffeine and may experience feelings of anxiety after consuming it. Studies show that caffeine can improve our energy levels and help us to feel less tired (Smith et al. 1993). But if you're using caffeine as a short-term fix to help boost low energy levels, it may be worth looking at your overall diet instead.

Whether or not consuming coffee is beneficial in general is something we get asked all the time (and have also dedicated a *Forking Wellness* podcast episode to).

The following is our summarisation of the research:

» Individuals often favour coffee because of its ability to boost mood and physical performance—and there's research to support this.

» Caffeine stimulates the nervous system and increases epinephrine (that adrenaline rush), which can reportedly improve physical performance. Based on this information, it's suggested that consuming a cup of coffee 30 minutes before a workout may help you feel more energised (Doherty and Smith 2004; Anderson and Hickey 1994; Doherty and Smith 2005).

» Research reports coffee drinkers to be at a decreased risk of developing type 2 diabetes, although it's unclear as to why this may be the case (Huxley et al. 2009).

» Coffee drinkers have also been linked to having a lower risk of suffering from Alzheimer's disease and Parkinson's disease (Maia and De Mendonça 2002; Ascherio et al. 2004).

» Coffee is actually a good source of antioxidants, which help prevent oxidative damage (Pulido, Hernandez-Garcia, and Saura-Calixto 2003).

Remember that no single food or drink guarantees good health, but it's helpful to know the research behind certain things—especially if you love your coffee. Now, if you don't love coffee, this by no means suggests you need to start drinking it—in fact, there's some research that's not so in favour of coffee. Some individuals simply don't react well to caffeine or to too much caffeine in their system and may experience feelings of anxiety, heart palpitations, or panic attacks (Winston, Hardwick, and Jaberi 2005). If this is the case for you, we recommend you opt for a lifestyle that limits caffeine intake. Too much caffeine can also disrupt sleep and affect sleep quality. We recommended cutting down on caffeine after noon, and if you do struggle with getting to sleep, try and wean yourself off the caffeine and see if it makes a difference.

Some people may even feel addicted to caffeine and feel like they can't function without it. If this is the case for you, you may suffer from withdrawal symptoms when you don't have it, such as headaches or brain fog. Decide if caffeine actually benefits your lifestyle and make an informed decision as to how often you want to drink it (Juliano and Griffiths 2004).

Our bodies are all so different, so it really is up to you to decide whether or not you think caffeine is worth it. Some of our clients enjoy it, and some don't—you do you!

# What About Intuitive Eating?

Disclaimer: This isn't an intuitive-eating-focused book, but we believe in a non-diet approach, so we've given a brief overview of what intuitive eating is as a starter guide.

## WHAT IS IT?

Intuitive Eating (IE) is a non-diet approach developed by registered dietitians Evelyn Tribole and Elyse Resch in the mid-1990s that intends to help individuals heal from chronic dieting. Diets come with a variety of side effects, such as slowed metabolism, disordered eating behaviours, feelings of guilt and anxiety regarding food, binge eating (usually as a result of restriction), and rebound weight gain. Learning how to eat intuitively can help individuals make rational food choices based on feelings of hunger, energy requirements, and preferences. When dieting, food choices often come with guilt and encourage you to choose what to eat based on the calorific value of the food. Imagine being able to listen to your hunger signals, respect your body's needs, and choose foods you actually want to eat. That's what IE helps you to achieve. It allows you to tune in to your body's internal messages and meet your psychological and biological needs. It strips away food rules and takes away the perceived positive and negative labels you've been associating with certain foods. For example, diet culture considers an apple good because it's low in calories and fat and a chocolate bar bad because it's high in sugar. IE encourages you to legalise all foods so you can instead look at specific food as a delicious part of your overall diet. All food is fit—some just contains more nutrients than others.

Think about your favourite food that you've associated with being off-limits or not allowed because you're on a diet or trying to lose weight. (Common foods in this category are chocolate, cake, and pizza). Now imagine if we told you that you were allowed to eat only that one food for a whole week or even just three days. How would you feel? You'd likely be craving balance—other foods like vegetables and proteins. By legalising all foods, the 'bad' ones lose their appeal. And you might actually end up enjoying that food when you genuinely feel like having it, and you won't be ridden with feelings of guilt.

| Consequences of Dieting | Things IE Has Been Associated With |
|---|---|
| » slowed metabolism | » improved body image |
| » disordered eating patterns | » improved metabolism |
| » feelings of guilt and anxiety regarding food and eating | » reduced levels of anxiety about food |
| » binge eating, usually as a result of restriction | » improved self-esteem |
| » rebound weight gain | » weight maintenance (not weight loss) |

## TEN PRINCIPLES OF IE

This is a very brief overview of the IE approach, and if you decide you need further guidance, there are plenty of resources in our reference list, and you may want to seek one-on-one nutrition support.

IE is in no way a diet, and there are no rules. But it's made up of 10 principles, which are here to guide you on your journey, at your own pace.

1. **Ditch the diets and reject diet mentality.** This first principle helps you to first address your own food rules—the rules that have meant you've categorised foods into 'good' and 'bad'—and secondly challenge them and get rid of them. Now, we know this is a lot easier said than done, but the more you fight them, the happier you'll ultimately be. It's important to be patient and remember that you might have years' worth of unlearning to do.

2. **Honour hunger.** Diets encourage you to ignore your hunger signals. In fact, we've worked with clients who've said they feel guilty when they feel hungry. But feeling hungry is a positive thing. It's your body's way of telling you it requires energy. But if you override those hunger pangs and restrict food, your body is likely to react with the urgency to binge. We need to be able to tune in to our hunger signals so we can respond. Note that some of us will take a while to feel again in tune with these signals, as a result of neglecting them. But don't worry, and remember to be patient with yourself.

3. **Make peace with food.** Once you start to challenge your negative thoughts regarding food, you can start to change the way you think about food and make peace with it. At this stage, you should give yourself unconditional permission to eat—and this doesn't mean you need to sit and binge on food. The idea here is that if you know you'll have access to all kinds of foods whenever you want them, food won't be so forbidden. Let's take a box of chocolates, for example. Diet mentality might think, If I eat them all tonight, I can start restricting again tomorrow. IE mentality will think, Eat as much as I'm comfortable with, and if I want another one, I can have one again when I truly feel like having one.

4. **Challenge the food police.** *The food* police tends to say things such as: You're 'good' for eating a salad for lunch and 'bad' for having a dessert. Fork that! These are unreasonable rules that have been created as a result of diet culture, however, they often pop up on a daily basis for those who've

been or are dieting. The food police might take a while to get rid of completely, and these thoughts will need to be challenged regularly.

5. **Respect your fullness.** This principle helps you to listen and tune in to your body's signals that inform you you're feeling satiated. Here are things that can help: pausing halfway through your meal and checking in with yourself: How does my body feel? Does the food taste good? How full am I feeling? Mindful eating can be helpful here, too (see page 78).

6. **Discover the satisfaction factor.** There's a difference between feeling full and feeling satisfied. When you eat what you really want and what your body is asking for, the feelings of pleasure and satisfaction should help you feel content. This often takes less food than we anticipate.

7. **Honour your feelings without using food.** The majority of us have experienced emotional eating. And there's nothing wrong with that. Emotional eating is normal, however, when we turn to this coping mechanism every time something goes wrong, it can become problematic. This principle crosses over with the next principle. Learn to respect yourself enough to look after your body in helpful ways. Create a list of things you can do to comfort yourself when you might otherwise turn to food for comfort. For example, take a bubble bath, read a book, go for a walk, journal. Keep this list and refer to it when you feel the urge to eat because you're emotional. Remember, eating to comfort yourself is fine, but having other tools to use is helpful too.

8. **Respect your body.** Accept body diversity. Most of us are guilty of judging ourselves. Learning to respect your body is extremely important. If you spend your time being critical of your body and can't accept the skin you live in, it becomes very hard to reject the diet mentality. If you're struggling with your body image and you find it getting in the way of your IE journey, psychological support may be necessary.

9. **Exercise—feel the difference.** Diet culture tells us that we have to exercise to burn off calories. This can be a very unenjoyable way of exercising and, furthermore, our bodies *need* food. Food doesn't need to be 'earned'. Movement can help you manage stress, improve cardiovascular health, lower blood pressure, and contribute to overall well-being—much more helpful reasons to encourage you to move your body. This principle helps you uncouple weight loss from exercise. Although it's possible to lose weight through exercise, that shouldn't be the intention. Your health should be your priority, and remember that BMI isn't representative of how healthy you are. Try doing an exercise you actually enjoy.

You don't have to run or do a High-Intensity Interval Training (HIIT) workout. You can dance, do a group workout, try a class with a friend, take your dog for a walk, or go swimming, for example. You may find it helpful to keep a movement journal documenting how your exercise affects your sleep, mood, and energy levels and also get rid of any tracking apps or watches.

10. **Gentle nutrition—honour your health.** Although this principle can be applied throughout your IE journey, it's the final principle as it's important for you to understand that food should be enjoyed as well as serve the purpose of supporting health.

## SO YOU WANT TO START IE—WHERE DO YOU BEGIN?

Diet culture has taught us that we can't trust our bodies. So starting your journey to eating intuitively can be pretty daunting because you've been listening to social and environmental factors instead of your own body. It's important to remember that IE is a journey and doesn't happen overnight. There are no rules, no 'blowing it', and no timeline you need to work within.

So if it weren't for diet culture and all the messages we've been bombarded with from a young age telling us that smaller bodies are more worthy, we might actually be pretty good at understanding what our bodies want and need and stop trying to shrink them. Know this: your weight is independent of your health. A lot of the time when we go on a diet, we tend to neglect our health. We can become so fixated on losing weight that nourishment seems to take a back seat. IE puts weight loss in the back seat instead. We all have individual set points, something that's explained more on page 89. The 10 principles don't have to be done in order, and we've put together the following helpful points with regard to starting your journey. This will help guide what actions may be best to take first if you are new to the concept of IE.

### Start Thinking About Your Food Choices
When deciding what to eat, try drowning out that 'devil' voice you've likely been listening to. You know, the one that's been telling you that you 'shouldn't' eat this and you 'can't' have that. Ask yourself, Are my food choices based on what I actually like and want, or am I listening to my inner critic? Am I choosing foods based on calorie or fat content? Identifying these thoughts and behaviours can help you tackle them. Try and think about the foods that are likely to truly satisfy you. There's a difference between feeling full and satisfied. For example, you want the chocolate bar, but you choose to have a low-calorie snack instead. You don't feel satisfied, so you have another one and another one—you probably should have just had the chocolate bar, eh? Try and choose foods your body is asking for instead of trying to avoid certain foods you later might find yourself bingeing on.

### Tell the Food Police to Fork Off!
As mentioned, exposure to diet culture formed the voice of the food police in your head. The misinformation you've heard gives you reason to question your body's needs. When you hear this voice, tell it to fork off. Additionally, we often find ourselves comparing what we're eating to what our friend, sister, mum, or boyfriend is eating, but why should that matter? Our bodies are all unique, which means our food choices should be too.

### Ditch the Scales

Is the first thing you do in the morning stepping on the scale? If the answer is yes, ask yourself if it enhances your life in a positive way. I'm going to guess and say your answer is likely to be a no. The scale can't possibly predict one's health. It's just a number. So why let it have so much power over you?

### Try Mindful Eating

We talk about this in detail on page 78, but we've both, in our personal lives and professional experience, known this to be very helpful when it comes to food appreciation. Research has associated mindful eating with increased food enjoyment and decreased episodes of bingeing (Masuda, Price, and Latzman 2012). It's also been suggested that it helps those who suffer from disordered eating patterns, depression, and anxiety (Kristeller and Wolever 2011).

## WHAT ARE THE BENEFITS OF IE?

This is an emerging area of research that's continuing to grow, however, it's important to note that the existing research is largely focused on women. Studies have demonstrated that IE is linked to healthier psychological attitudes, and although not a weight loss tool, it's been associated with weight maintenance (Van Dyke and Drinkwater 2014).

Individuals who've taken part in IE studies have also shown improved self-esteem, better body image, and reduced symptoms of stress and anxiety (Schaefer and Magnuson 2014). They're also less likely to demonstrate disordered eating habits (Bruce and Ricciardelli 2016).

Not only has IE been shown to improve overall well-being, but studies have demonstrated good retention rates (Schaefer and Magnuson 2014). Unlike diets, IE encourages sustainable behaviours, and people are more likely to keep practising the positive changes they've made. Diets, on the other hand, tend to be short-lived and often result in weight gain in the long run.

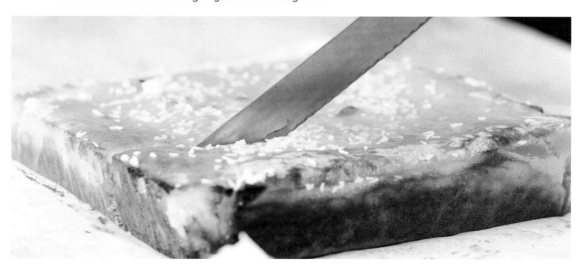

## HUNGER SIGNALS: LEARNING TO LISTEN TO AND UNDERSTAND YOUR BODY'S SIGNALS

Googling what to eat and when to eat it can lead you to mistrust your own internal signals. The truth is, our bodies are pretty clever. We have specific hormones for specific functions, and those include letting us know when we're hungry. What should be an intuitive process is often disturbed by—yep, you guessed it—diet culture. A lot of us will at some point need to relearn to trust our bodies. The first step towards doing this is understanding the difference between physical and emotional hunger.

| Physical Hunger | Emotional Hunger |
|---|---|
| Physical hunger is your biological need for food | Emotional Hunger is driven by emotions |
| Signs of physical hunger include low energy, irritability, stomach rumbles, growing hunger pangs, significant time having passed since you last ate, and food being satisfying once eaten. | Signs of emotional hunger include specific cravings—such as chocolate or cake (known as comfort foods), finding yourself wandering around the kitchen looking for food, being frustrated and feeling you need to turn to food, and it not being long ago that you last ate. |

Albers 2009.

Ghrelin, known as the 'hunger hormone', is produced in the gut and signals the brain when it's time to eat (Klok, Jakobsdottir, and Drent 2007). Its levels increase, and we feel hungry, which usually means the body requires more food. Ghrelin is released into the bloodstream, signalling the brain that it's time to eat, and decreases when the stomach starts to feel full (Cummings et al. 2001). Leptin (the 'satiety hormone') signals to us that we're full or have had enough food. If you've ever been on a diet, you've likely ignored these signals at some point, whether it be eating less than you needed or overeating because you felt restricted. It may take some time to identify with these signals again.

# INTUITIVE EATING FAQS

1. **Will I lose weight?**
   IE isn't a diet, and we encourage you to turn your focus away from any weight-related goal and accept that your days of dieting are over. We want you to want to focus on your overall health and well-being and to realise that weight and health are two different things. We're all born different shapes and sizes, and although IE may result in some weight loss, good overall health is more important.

2. **How long does it take?**
   There's no set time frame in which you can expect to feel like you've mastered IE, and unlike diets, it's not a quick fix. IE is a journey, and it may take some people longer, depending on how many years they may have been battling a disordered or dysfunctional relationship with food. Some individuals may find it helpful to have psychological support throughout their journey too.

3. **How do I know if I'm actually hungry?**
   Those who have a long history of dieting are likely to find themselves questioning what actual hunger feels like and will be disconnected from their hunger and satiety signals. There are a few things you can do to identify if you're hungry, but also know that as time goes on and you start to eat 'normally' again, these signals may become more apparent. Firstly, ask yourself, On a scale of 1 to 10 (1 being painfully hungry, and 10 being painfully full), where do I land? sit? You can also use the previous physical-hunger–emotional-hunger table.

4. **What if all I want to eat are 'unhealthy' foods?**
   Initially, you might feel a little out of control. Remember that bingeing is often a result of restriction, so if all you want to do is eat cake, maybe it's worth getting that out of your system. Let's put it this way: imagine if you were allowed to eat only cake for five days straight—the novelty would likely wear off pretty quickly, and you'd be craving something a little more balanced.

5. **Can you eat intuitively when you have or have had an ED?**
   This very much depends on what stage you're at in terms of recovery. Meal plans are often necessary in the initial treatment of an ED in order to help renourish the body, and individuals should work closely with both a dietitian and some form of psychological support. But this isn't to say you can't start to adopt some of the principles, such as rejecting the diet mentality and respecting your body. We're all unique and work at different paces, so don't feel discouraged if you've been told you're not 'ready' to practice IE. As mentioned, you can still start to work on some of the principles but also accept that recovery takes time and that weight restoration will likely need to be prioritised.

6. **I have a medical condition—will IE work for me?**
   It's very possible to eat intuitively alongside an existing or diagnosed medical condition, however, you may need additional guidance. We'd advise working with a non-diet clinician to address any dietary needs, which can include IBS, high cholesterol, and polycystic ovarian syndrome (PCOS). IE is about getting to know your body and respecting what it needs, so this can apply to anyone.

# Eating Behaviours

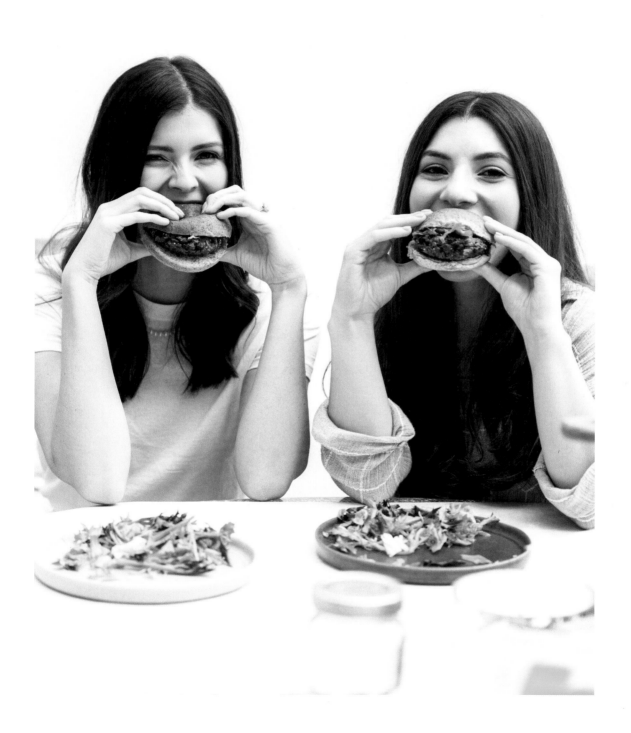

# Mindfulness: Tips for Mindful Eating

Mindful eating can be considered a form of meditation, and it can help you acknowledge your eating experience. It may sound time-consuming, but there's some convincing research behind the concept, and on an anecdotal note, we've both experienced positive outcomes with the approach, both with clients and personally. It teaches you to use your senses to identify what foods truly satisfy you as well as leave you feeling nourished. It may also help you become more in tune with your hunger and satiety signals. If you have a habit of identifying foods in a negative way and judging your own food choices, this technique may also help neutralise those tendencies. Although not everyone will appreciate mindful eating, research suggests that it may be a helpful tool for a number of reasons:

» It's been associated with increased feelings of enjoyment whilst eating.

» It may help reduce episodes of bingeing.

» It may be helpful for individuals who suffer from EDs, depression, or anxiety.

There's no right or wrong way to eat, but choosing what to eat is something that some people find difficult to enjoy. In fact, you might be someone who finds it confusing, stressful, or anxiety provoking. Accept that everyone's eating experience is different, but whatever your habits, you deserve to enjoy mealtimes, and it's worth exploring ways that can help you do that.

Mindful eating involves the following:

» slowing down the rate in which you eat

» eating with little or no distractions

» tuning in to your physical hunger cues and distinguishing nonhunger triggers for eating

» using your senses to enhance your eating experience (e.g. smell, taste, touch)

» identifying and coping with guilt and anxiety regarding food

» eating to help maintain good well-being

» appreciating and enjoying food

It's unrealistic to prioritise mindful eating at each meal, because lots of people lead pretty busy lives. But try and incorporate this where and when you can, and it'll likely begin to feel more natural, and you may find yourself practising it more often than not. Start slow, and try it for at least one meal per week to begin with.

*Top Tip to Begin Experimenting With Mindful-Eating Practice*

» **Make a conscious effort to slow down the rate in which you chew your food.**

» **Chew thoroughly.**

» **Eliminate distractions (e.g. turning off the TV and putting down your phone).**

» **Try eating in silence or just have music on in the background if you prefer some background noise.**

» **Focus on how the food makes you feel.**

» **Focus on the taste and texture of the food.**

» **Savour each bite.**

» **Try and identify when you start to feel full.**

(Masuda, Price, and Latzman 2012; Kristeller and Wolever 2011; Grossman et al. 2004)

# Binge Eating

We want to touch on binge-eating disorder (BED) because the term binge has become so common in today's society. Even having the word used in phrases such as 'binge-watch a Netflix series' takes the severity out of its true meaning. We often hear individuals use the term binge in sentences such as these: 'I totally binged on biscuits last night. I had about eight digestives.' or 'I binged last night and ate a whole bag of sweets.'

Well, we're here to say these are definitely not clinical binges but rather instances of overeating—there is a difference. But this does highlight how subjective the term is. Remember, one person's binge could be another's usual mid-afternoon snack. And with the subjectivity of the word binge also comes the misuse of the BED diagnosis.

To understand what BED and a clinical binge entails, refer to the DSM-5 criteria in the following list.

## DSM-5 Diagnostic Criteria for BED**

» **Criterion 1: Recurrent episodes of binge eating characterised by both of the following:**

   » **Eating, in a discrete period of time (e.g., within any two-hour period), an amount of food that is definitely larger than most people would eat in a similar period under similar circumstances**

   » **Sense of a lack of control over eating during the episode (e.g., a feeling that one cannot stop eating or control what or how much on is eating)**

» **Criterion 2: Binge-eating episodes are associated with three (or more) of the following:**

   » **Eating much more rapidly than normal**

   » **Eating until feeling uncomfortably full**

   » **Eating large amounts of food when not feeling physically hungry**

   » **Eating alone because of being embarrassed by how much one is eating**

   » **Feeling disgusted with oneself, depressed, or very guilty after overeating**

» **Criterion 3: Marked distress regarding binge eating is present.**

» **Criterion 4: Binge eating occurs, on average, at least one day/week for three months.**

» **Criterion 5: Binge eating is not associated with regular use of inappropriate compensatory behaviors (e.g. purging, fasting, excessive exercise) and does not occur exclusively during the course of anorexia nervosa or bulimia nervosa.**

*If you feel you identify with these criteria, please make an appointment to talk to your GP at the earliest convenience or visit http://beateatingdisorders.org.uk.

**Vahia 2013.

As of 2013, the American Psychiatric Association characterises BED as an ED, ultimately classifying it as a mental-health disorder. But when most people hear the words *eating disorder*, they associate images of underweight individuals or people who 'look sick'. But BED is actually the most common ED because it affects roughly 3 percent of the population, which is huge when compared with the 0.4 percent prevalence of anorexia nervosa (Brownley et al. 2016).

So if BED is the most common ED, why is it not often spoken about?

Well, sadly, we believe that most people overlook BED for several reasons. Firstly, it was only recently added to the *DSM-5*, so it's fairly new, and many may not even know it exists. But, the lack of conversation around BED is most likely due to the stigmas associated with it. As individuals with BED are more likely to be overweight or obese, some may not perceive them to 'fit the part' of someone with an ED, aesthetically speaking. Plus the guilt and shame that are entangled with BED and obesity lead to a lack of awareness and advocacy. But not all overweight individuals suffer from BED, and not all individuals with BED are overweight, which makes it difficult to understand, because it's not always obvious to spot someone who's suffering (which is the case for many mental-health conditions).

BED is quite a complex condition, and while we don't want to spend too much time discussing it as this isn't a book about EDs, we think it's imperative we mention a few key things:

» Genetic, environmental, family, and social factors all contribute to the development of BED.

» Having a larger body during childhood and adolescence increases vulnerability to the disorder.

» Exposure to emotional eating, restrictive eating (especially in the family), body dissatisfaction, dieting, and an internalised 'thin ideal' also increase the risk for development of BED.

» A large portion of the research supports that binges correlate with negative affect and difficulty regulating emotions.

» BED is usually associated with other psychiatric disorders, most commonly depression.

» The primary treatments for BED include psychological and behavioural therapies, such as cognitive behavioural therapy (CBT), not nutrition-focused treatment.

» Pharmacology (medicine) is often involved in treatment.

» Approximately 50 percent of patients still remain symptomatic post-treatment. (Kornstein et al. 2016; Lewer et al. 2017; Burton and Abbott 2019; Stice and Burger 2015)

We hope this list highlights that a true BED diagnosis is a psychiatric condition and requires the appropriate treatment, whether that's therapy, medication, or both. The lines can be quite blurred with BED because it centres around food. But as nutrition professionals, we feel the strong need to highlight that BED isn't a nutrition-related condition nor should it be treated solely by a registered dietitian or registered nutritionist.

## EMOTIONAL EATING

Non-BED binges are very common. Personally, both of us can admit we occasionally binge—not sure if other health professionals are so quick to admit this, but just remember, we're regular people. In fact, we can guarantee both of us have turned to food while writing this book. (It's been very stressful at times . . .)

Emotional eating can be a helpful coping strategy. Food provides comfort—it tastes good, it makes us happy, and a particular food may be tied to certain events or past experiences that offer solace. For example, if your mum always made you buttered toast when you were feeling unwell, you may associate it with your mum's care or comfort—which may lead you to turn towards this option when experiencing moments of insecurity or self-doubt.

The problem with using food as a means to cope with your emotions arises when it's the only coping strategy you have. At the end of this chapter, we'll discuss some alternative coping strategies and tools. But for now, we just want you to understand the following:

*Binge* is a subjective term.

» The occasional binge doesn't mean you have BED.

» The occasional binge isn't a bad thing, and it's actually really normal.

» Having alternative coping strategies is important.

Now, what about the binge-restrict cycle? After restricting yourself, you will feel empty and overly hungry. Then you will begin to have obsessive thoughts around food; you start to eat. At this point, you begin to binge. You might start to feel guilty and out of control, so then you feel the need to 'make up for it' or somehow regain your control. You then restrict yourself, and the binge-restrict cycle begins again.

You may recognise this cycle. The theory is pretty straightforward and is comprised of four steps:

1. **You restrict your food for a particular reason.** Maybe you're following a certain diet that has a banned-food list. Maybe you cut out carbs in an attempt to lose weight quickly or you tell yourself you're 'being good' and have sworn off cakes, biscuits, chocolate, etc. Whatever your restriction may be, you've told yourself certain foods are off-limits and you're not allowed to have them.

2. **You start to eat (start to binge).** The tension has built up, and you can no longer take it. The biscuits are in front of you. You told yourself you wouldn't eat them anymore, but they look so tempting. You may even think to yourself, Let me eat as much as I can right now because after this I'll never have them again. Or you might think, I've already failed—I might as well just have all the biscuits.

3. **The guilt hits.** Once the act of bingeing is over, you may ask yourself, Why the fork did I just do that? The guilt, shame, regret, and feelings of worthlessness kick in. You may even feel physically sick, thirsty, nauseous, or uncomfortable.

4. **But it's 'OK'—you have a newfound resolution to 'never do this again'.** In fact, you may feel so disgusted or upset that the only way to right this 'wrong' is to restrict this food once more. You may think, Look what just happened—clearly I can't be trusted around this food.

Can you relate?

Yeah? Same.

Remember, it *is* OK. But have a look at the diagram again. Now, remove the restriction. Viola! (You can thank us later, ha ha!)

But seriously, if we remove the restriction, we can break the cycle. It's human instinct to want the things we can't have and to break rules. (Rules are meant to be broken, right?) Think back to when you were younger. If your mum or dad said, 'You can't have this', didn't it make you want it more? Or if you tell a kid, 'Don't touch that', what do you think they do the moment you turn around?

Well, based on clinical observations and animal studies, scientists have identified that dieting and restrictive eating are driving forces for binge eating (Stice and Burger 2015). Furthermore, there's a growing body of evidence that supports the idea that there's a causal link from dietary restriction to bingeing. Now, we can't say that if you restrict your

Remember, a single binge doesn't equate to BED, and only medics can diagnose.

food choices you'll binge. And not all BED cases stem from restriction. Remember, BED involves recurrent and frequent binges preceded by distress or depression (negative affects) and the act of bingeing is used to cope with these emotions. But we can say that restriction (and dieting) increases our risk for binges and developing BED, which, as we discussed, is an eating disorder. Just another reason to ditch the forking diets.

## Minnesota Starvation Experiment*

Now, if you've read any other anti-diet books, we can guarantee you've heard about this before. But for those who are new to the anti-diet research, or genuinely find the research interesting (like us), let's discuss this unique moment in history.

Let's set the scene:

It was 1944, and thanks to World War II, several populations were in crisis of starvation. And Ancel Keys, a PhD at the Laboratory of Physiological Hygiene at the University of Minnesota, and Josef Brozek, a PhD from Charles University (Prague), were eager to study the physiological and psychological effects of starvation. They designed the Minnesota Starvation Experiment, a study for which 36 young men volunteered. It's important to note that all 36 men were single and demonstrated good physical and mental health (amongst other criteria).

The research protocol was as follows:

» The men had to lose 25 percent of their pre-study weight. (None of them were overweight to start.)

» In the first three months, they consumed a normal diet of 3,200 calories per day.

» During the next six months, their daily calorie intake was cut by more than half, amounting to 1,570 and divided between two meals (a semi-starvation state).

» Following that, the men entered a three-month restricted rehabilitation period, where the men could consume 2,000–3,200 calories a day.

» The final eight weeks consisted of unrestricted rehab, where the men had full control on how much they ate.

» During the study, the men were required to work 15 hours per week, walk 22 miles per week, and participate in educational activities for 25 hours per week.

The main takeaways from the study include the following:

» During the starvation period, the men demonstrated significant decreases in strength, stamina, core body temperature, heart rate, and sex drive.

» Hunger resulted in feelings of obsession with regard to food. They dreamt, fantasised, talked, and read about food.

» The men reported feeling tired, irritable, depressed, and apathetic. They also reported feelings of decreased mental ability, although their test scores reflected otherwise.

» During the unrestricted rehabilitation period most men engaged in extreme overeating.

» For many, the preoccupation and obsession with food lingered despite weight restoration.

*Baker and Keramidas 2013.

Before we move on to the next chapter, we want to reiterate that not all episodes of emotional eating are binges. While occasional binges are completely normal, if you do find yourself turning to food to cope with emotions more commonly than not, we highly recommend you speak to your GP or make an appointment with a psychologist. If you're diagnosed with BED, remember, it's a psychology-related matter, not a nutrition-related matter. Working with a registered dietitian or registered nutritionist alongside a psychologist may be helpful, but working exclusively with a dietitian or nutritionist isn't advised.

## Forking Wellness Takeaways

Restriction (even for just three months) can have harmful effects, both physiological and psychological. Intentional restriction can also have long-term effects, such as continued preoccupation or obsession with food and extreme overeating. Restriction of any type should be avoided—unless medically necessary, of course (Stice and Burger 2015).

So if you find yourself using food as an occasional coping strategy, it's OK. But it's imperative to have a multitude of strategies to help deal with your emotions and to prevent future episodes of emotionally overeating.

Here are a few strategies and tools that we—yes, we—use:

» Prioritise balanced meals. Ensuring we have a good balance of nutrients (carbohydrates, protein, fat, and fibre) at most meals can help us prevent feeling deprived or ravenous, both of which can lead to overeating at future meals.

» **Remove all the rules.** Remember, restriction results in feelings of deprivation, which lead us to enter the binge-restrict cycle. (Refer back to the 'What About Intuitive Eating?' chapter for more information on this.)

» **Ensure satisfaction.** While you opt for a certain meal because it's balanced, it might not be satisfying. If you're missing the satisfaction factor, you may find you have lingering cravings. If you're craving pizza, a salad just isn't going to cut it.

» **Practise mindfulness.** Mindfulness strategies have been used to help treat emotional dysregulation. Slowing down and checking in with your surroundings, senses, thoughts, feelings, and environment can help you make rational decisions. Additionally, research suggests that mindfulness meditations can help decrease binges and emotional eating (Barney et al. 2019; Katterman et al. 2014). (Refer to the section on mindfulness for more information.)

» **Find a distraction method that works for you.** If you're feeling emotional discomfort, choose a non-food-related form of distraction. For Bari, this includes knitting or completing a sudoku puzzle. For Sophie, this includes doing a full-body stretch or listening to a podcast (we obviously recommend the Forking Wellness podcast) while walking her dog, Bear.

» **Journal.** It's easy to let thoughts build up in your head. Over time, they can become increasingly loud and not very kind. Putting pen to paper helps to emotionally digest these thoughts and reflect upon them. Additionally, transferring any negative thoughts from your mind to a piece of paper can symbolically mean they're no longer your thoughts.

» **Talk to someone.** We don't mean just friends or family. While having friends and family to lean on for emotional support is important, talking to a professional is invaluable. We highly recommend therapy for those who can afford it.

» **Don't dwell on the past.** The past is in the past—literally. Remember, you always have the ability to choose your next move. You're not bound by the previous decisions you've made. But reflecting on past experiences can be a positive opportunity for growth. You might ask yourself this: Next time, how would I handle this situation differently?

# What the Fork Is Willpower?

Seriously, what the fork is willpower? Is it something we're born with, or is it a learned trait? Why do some people have it and others not?

Although *willpower* refers to your ability to control your emotions, actions, or urges, using this term in the context of dieting poses a problem (*Merriam-Webster* 2003). In diet context, a lack of willpower refers to an inherent fault in one's personality. In other words, some might associate having a piece of chocolate cake with 'lack of willpower'. That can further spirals someone into guilt and shame for not being 'strong' enough, which results in the following illogical conclusion: The act of having a piece of chocolate cake means I'm weak. I've done something wrong; therefore, I should be punished. The act of going against my moral compass means I feel guilty and ashamed, maybe even punished.

All of these emotions for having a slice of cake? Uh . . . thank you—next?

The concept of willpower, or lack thereof, in the context of eating is a product of diet culture. The industry tactfully plays on this idea to keep you paying for products and new diets. If your willpower is always failing you, you'll always want to be on a diet. And who benefits if you're always on a diet? Well, the diet-and-weight-loss industry, of course.

> The diet-and-weight-loss industry sets you up to fail, which leaves you thinking, It's not you—it's me. But we—Bari and Sophie—are here to say, it's not you—it's the forking diet's fault!

Here's our *Forking Wellness* guide to why willpower doesn't exist in terms of dieting and health:

**The rules are too strict.** We've already touched on this concept, but the reason you give into 'temptation' isn't because you lack self-control; it's because the rules are too restrictive and unrealistic. If you swear off sugar in an attempt to lose weight or improve your health, your self-restraint has a finite capacity. You might pass up your first piece of chocolate, but can you do this forever? Absolutely not. And who'd want to! Refer back to the binge-restrict cycle if you want to explore this problem further, but remember, willpower in terms of food behaviours is just a guise for restriction.

**Cravings are normal.** Not all cravings are created equal. Sometimes we crave a bag of crisps, and other times, we crave a salad. Why should giving in to a 'healthy' craving be deemed as listening to your body but giving in to an 'unhealthy' craving means lack of willpower? Unfortunately, giving in to your cravings has earned a bad reputation. While we already discussed the importance of listening to your body (see the 'What About Intuitive Eating?' chapter) and how this can improve your relationship with food, the concept of willpower has undermined a natural and healthy decision-making skill. We all have cravings, and they should all be honoured, because if you don't honour them, you'll continue to seek out satisfaction in other ways.

**There's a difference between intrinsic vs. extrinsic motivation.** The type of motivation you have for making (or not making) a particular decision can predict the outcome. In this context, there are two types of motivation: intrinsic and extrinsic. *Intrinsic motivation* refers to doing something because you want to—it makes you feel good. For example, you might be motivated to go to a yoga class because you know you always feel calmer when you leave and your muscles feel nice and stretched. On the other hand, *extrinsic motivation* refers to the motivation to perform (or not perform) an act based on a reward or consequence. For example, you may be extrinsically motivated to post on Instagram to get more likes or show up to work to get paid. Basic, but true. (Benabou and Tirole 2003).

**Decisions require both types of motivation.** We need a balance of the two types of motivation to make sustained, ongoing decisions. Willpower, in terms of diet, appeals to only extrinsic motivations. In other words, you may avoid the piece of cake because you fear it'll have a negative consequence, such as weight gain (an extrinsic motivator). But you intrinsically want the piece of cake because you enjoy the taste. This disconnect between intrinsic and extrinsic motivation results in decisions to disobey the extrinsic motivator (willpower). Your actions aren't due to a lack of willpower—they're due to a lack of intrinsic motivation, because you don't really want to avoid the cake.

# Let's Be Real

# Set Point

If you're someone who's been yo-yo dieting for most of your life, you may be at the point where you're questioning if something is wrong with you and wondering why, despite the restrictive lifestyle, you're not reaching or maintaining your weight-loss goal. In this chapter, we aim to help you better understand the body and how it reacts when you restrict food intake.

When you go on a diet (any kind of diet), you're likely to lose weight. But with that comes many other consequences. Often it's thought that our body shapes are simply dependent on the type of diet we have, however, how we look is heavily determined by genetic factors, with environmental factors playing a role too (Müller, Bosy-Westphal, and Heymsfield 2010). As individuals, we have something called a set point—a weight range in

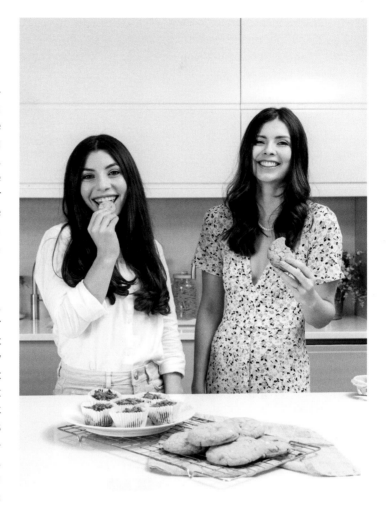

which one's body sits comfortably, can be flexible and nonrestrictive about food, doesn't feel the need to overeat regularly, and functions optimally day-to-day.

It's important, however, to note that your set point can fluctuate by a few pounds, and we as professionals don't recommend weighing yourself as there are many factors that can influence your weight that may not be representative of body fat.

We all have different set points, which is why if we ate the same amounts of food as each other, we'd never have the same-looking body, because genetically we're unique. There's been convincing research to support evidence that tells us that the majority of people who lose weight through dieting will put it back on—plus excess weight (Wolpert 2007). When you go on a diet, your body is actually fighting to get back to its set point, which is why some people who are trying to fight their weight will feel like they are in a constant struggle. This might not be the answer you were looking for, but trust us, getting to know and understand your body will lead to a much healthier and happier life than fighting your weight for the rest of your days. You'll do well to love and accept your body for all it does for you, and if you're living in a healthy body, be grateful for that. We're not expecting you to suddenly love your body overnight, and judging by our personal experience, no matter what size you are, you'll always have things you want to change about your body. But if you notice yourself speaking negatively about your appearance, hopefully the following table can help.

| Instead of . . . | Try . . . |
|---|---|
| My legs are so big. | My legs carry me around and enable me to do day-to-day activities. |
| I hate the shape of my tummy. | My health is the most important thing. |
| I wish I weighed less. | I'm so much more than the number on the scale. |

To put it simply, when you restrict your overall calorie intake, your body's metabolism slows down in response to less energy, meaning you need less food to maintain your weight. You feel less energised and crave more food. You eat more, and you put on weight again. If you're trying to recover from chronic dieting, you need to give your body time to readjust. As we've touched on previously, this may mean eating more than you're used to for a while.

# Body Neutrality

With the rise of the body-positive movement (which we're totally all for, by the way), we can't help but think we need to address the fact that the idea of 'loving your body' may feel a little overwhelming for some. Now, we're no experts in this area of emerging research, but we want to do a bit of an overview so you can feel a little more educated on the subject and hopefully start to learn to love your body or at least feel less negatively towards it.

| Body Positivity | Body Neutrality |
|---|---|
| This is the idea that regardless of your size, shape, and appearance, you should feel positive towards yourself | This steers you away from hating your appearance and spending too much energy thinking about your bodies in a negative way. |

Beyond being what we look like, our bodies do amazing things for us. They keep us breathing, carry us, support us physically and mentally, and allow us to bond and create relationships with people—which is what life is all about, right? Unfortunately, diet culture encourages us to become fixated on what we look like, like it's the most important thing in the world. But it's not. It's the least important. What matters is who you are, what you stand for, who you love, how you care for people, and how you look after yourself in a positive way to support your mental health. What do you want people to remember you for—how much you weighed or what you were like as a person? (We're hoping you didn't go with 'how much you weighed'!) What we're trying to say is that wellness is about the happiness and health that come from the inside. What you look like doesn't determine how healthy you are. If you struggle with your body image, we suggest you seek qualified psychological support.

## DO WHAT YOU LOVE. LOVE WHAT YOU DO.

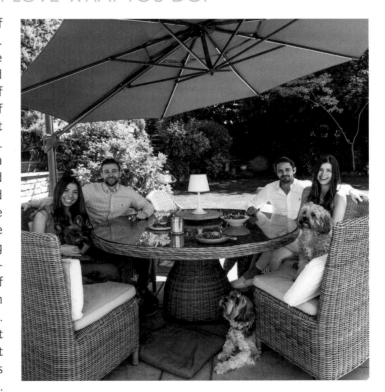

If you love chocolate, eat it. If you hate broccoli, don't eat it. Something we're both passionate about is helping individuals find their own unique definition of *wellness*, and we've seen a lot of people try and go against what their body feels comfortable doing. This is often fuelled by social media too. Remember when we were asked to believe that superfoods would magically make us healthy? Like those really expensive powders were the answers we'd all been looking for. As if health is that simple. Well-being is complex and made up of so many different factors (which we've been through in this book). You could have the healthiest diet (whatever that may look like) but also smoke, drink excessive amounts of alcohol, and suffer from insomnia.

Or you could eat your vegetables but also enjoy a slice of cake, sleep relatively well, and go running three times a week. The second option sounds a little more balanced, right? What we're trying to say is that any extreme behaviours likely won't get you where you've convinced yourself they will. It's what you do consistently over time that matters. Of course, if you eat only cake, you're not going to feel very healthy, but the same goes for vegetables. If you ate only fruit and veg all week, you'd probably feel awful. Try and take a step back and ask yourself what brings you enjoyment. Take weight out of the equation and think about how what you do makes you feel.

## SELF-CARE

*Self-care* seems to have been a bit of a buzzword over the past few years and may have left us feeling a little confused with regard to what it actually is. Self-care is defined as 'the practice of taking an active role in protecting one's own well-being and happiness'. And that means what?

Diet, sleep, and exercise are often the elements that come to mind when the word *self-care* is brought up. And whilst these are all important, what about actual relaxation or time out, away from thinking about food or how much movement you've done that day? Making sure you're satisfied and nourished, enabling your body to feel good through movement, and having a consistent sleeping pattern are all essential to looking after yourself. But self-care might also be about getting your nails done, spending quality time with a loved one, reading a book, taking a candle-lit bath—see where we're going with this? We believe it can be beneficial to make a conscious effort to do specific activities (often) that make you feel like you're looking after yourself—mind and body!

We've put together a self-care tool kit to help you figure out what your version of self-care looks like and how to prioritise it.

### Top Tips

- » **Put your phone down.**
- » **Get some fresh air.**
- » **Journal.**
- » **Take 20 minutes a day to do something for you. (This could even be just sitting in silence with your thoughts.)**

Your version of self-care is unique to you, and it can be really helpful to understand what this means to you so you can start to practise things that actually enhance your well-being—mentally and physically.

# Creating New Habits

So let's talk about habits! We've discussed things like focusing on balance, self-care, mindfulness, stress management, and good sleep routines and the importance of movement and nutrition, but how the fork do we actually implement these into our daily routines?

Change doesn't happen overnight, especially sustainable change. We know that if your diet 'starts on Monday', you may have to follow a new set of rules you're not used to. Overnight, you're expected to go from someone who eats porridge for breakfast to someone who's trying to cut down on carbs. Firstly, please don't feel like you can't have porridge for breakfast—we love porridge (especially with peanut butter). Second, conceptualising this idea in terms of a non-food-related habit may be easier to digest (pun intended). For example, if you've never run a day in your life, it's unlikely you'll wake up every morning at six and go for a 30-minute run before work. Even if you do it for a week, this routine may disappear as quickly as you initiated it. Becoming a person who runs before work sounds great, maybe even ideal. But let's back up a few steps and discuss how we can make this change a sustainable habit.

Let's start by defining *habit*. According to James Clear (2018), author of *Atomic Habits*, 'Habits are the small decisions you make and actions you perform every day. According to researchers at Duke University, habits account for about 40 percent of our behaviours on any given day. Your life today is essentially the sum of your habits'. We love this definition because it truly puts into perspective how influential our daily and unconscious decisions are. For example, brushing your teeth every night before bed and every morning before you leave the house is a habit. And without this habit, you may develop bad breath, rotting teeth, or mouth disease. Another habit may be as simple as getting into bed and setting your alarm on your phone for the following morning. You know if you don't set your alarm, you're likely to oversleep, causing you to be late for work.

> We highly recommend reading Atomic Habits. It's revolutionary!

Both these examples are positive habits. In other words, these actions lead to better outcomes, such as good oral hygiene and arriving to work on time, respectively. But negative habits can also exist. For example, you may go to sleep each night with your makeup on. When you wake up, you always seem to have a new breakout because your pores were clogged overnight. Or you scroll on Instagram for an hour before bed, which impairs your melatonin levels, resulting in a poor night's sleep.

As we said before, your identity lies within your habits, both good and bad. So how do we build positive and healthy habits and reduce our negative habits? First, let's break down the four stages of habits, as identified by Clear (2018).

1.  **Trigger:** Sometimes referred to as the cue, this is the action, thought, or situation that prompts a specific behaviour.

2.  **Motivation:** This is the desire to perform (or not perform) a certain act based on a trigger. You're motivated to make the decision for the perceived outcome or consequence.

3.  **Response:** This stage is the actual habit performed. The response isn't always an action—it could be a thought or feeling.

4.  **Reward:** The reward is what we want to achieve (or feel). Basically, the reward is the 'why' to the habit in the first place, which is essentially the satisfaction of the motivation. In other words, without the reward, what's the point?

Now that we've explained how habits work, we're going to walk you through our—Bari's and Sophie's—personal habits, both positive and negative.

| Positive Habit | | | | |
|---|---|---|---|---|
| Habit | Trigger | Motivation | Response | Reward |
| stretches for at least 10 minutes a day (Sophie) | waking up | wants to move body after a night's sleep because it feels good | stretches for 10 minutes on yoga mat | avoids feeling achy or stiff and body feels energised |
| brings a packed lunch to work every day (Bari) | cooking dinner the night before | doesn't have to spend money on buying lunch and wants to have a balanced meal | cooks an extra serving of dinner | saves money and has a delicious and balanced lunch |
| Negative Habits | | | | |
| Habit | Trigger | Motivation | Response | Reward |
| picks cuticles (Sophie) | feeling stressed or anxious | needs to exert some form of control in the situation | picks nails and cuticles | momentarily feels in control of the situation<br><br>consequence: sometimes has red and puffy cuticles |
| drinks coffee in the afternoon (Bari) | feeling tired or unmotivated around 3 p.m. | desires to feel alert and increase productivity | makes a cup of coffee | temporarily feels alert and motivated to tackle the afternoon to-do list<br><br>consequence: potential disruption to quality of sleep |

Next, we're going to walk you through how we plan to change our negative habits. (Hopefully, by the time you read this, we'll have accomplished this!) Remember, everyone is different, and we're all unique. But a helpful strategy is to replace a bad habit with an alternative action. In this instance, your trigger will remain the same, but your motivations, response, and reward will be different. In our case, the differences are motivated by the negative consequences accompanying our current 'rewards'. Some consider this an outcome-driven habit (de Wit et al. 2018). The following table provides examples:

| Changing Negative Habits | | | | |
|---|---|---|---|---|
| | Trigger | Motivation | New Habit/ Response | Reward |
| (Sophie) | feeling stressed or anxious | needs to exert some form of control in the situation plus maintain manicured fingers | takes a deep breath and writes down three positive actions to take to feel less stressed or less anxious | feels in control and proactive with regard to managing stress or anxiety and satisfied for not picking cuticles |
| (Bari) | feeling tired or unmotivated around 3 p.m. | desires to feel alert and increase productivity without compromising quality of sleep | decides to take a 10-minute walk outside | feels alert and motivated to tackle the afternoon to-do list and pleased about not making a cup of coffee |

But what about creating new habits?

We're glad you asked! When it comes to creating new habits, sometimes you have to reidentify the trigger or create your own. For example, here are some healthy habits we're personally working on:

| Creating New Habits | | | | |
|---|---|---|---|---|
| Habit | Trigger | Motivation | Response | Reward |
| attend at least one group exercise class per week (Sophie) | setting an alarm on Monday morning to sign up for a gym class | desires to increase fitness level in a group-based class because it's a more positive experience | uses a booking app to prepay for the class in advance and records the class in calendar | leaves the class feeling accomplished and positive while improving overall fitness |
| drink 2 L water every day (Bari) | bringing a 500 mL reusable water bottle everywhere | wants to prevent dehydration and promote overall health (especially skin appearance) | drinks four water-bottle equivalents each day (two before lunch and two after lunch) | is adequately hydrated and improving overall health (plus adding in extra daily steps from walking to and from the bathroom) |

When it comes to developing new habits, research suggests that visual triggers are often the most influential (Gardner, Lally, and Wardle 2012). Let's take the example of drinking more water. Carrying a reusable water bottle with you provides a visual reminder to drink more. Plus, you can physically feel if the bottom is empty (cue to fill it up) or full (cue to drink more).

On the other hand, hiding your triggers to negative habits can also be helpful. For example, let's say you're writing a book and your publisher has given you a strict deadline (hmm . . .). A bad habit you develop during this time might be using your phone as a form of procrastination (who, us?). But simply placing your phone in another room removes the potential for you to turn to this negative habit. By hiding the trigger, you can hide the habit.

> I (Bari) have found that placing my water bottle on my desk first thing in the morning is a really helpful reminder to drink more water. I also purchased a very brightly coloured (and slightly obnoxious) water bottle in an effort to have it continuously catch my eye. It's definitely helped me increase my overall fluids.

## SMALL HABITS SNOWBALL INTO BIGGER SHIFTS

Let's go back to our example of wanting to go on a 30-minute run every morning before work. We mentioned that change doesn't happen overnight and you can't expect your identity to change in a few hours. But by starting with a smaller habit, you're slowly putting one foot in front of the other towards building up to that habit. Remember, building healthy habits isn't a race. While they can improve your health over time, slow and steady change remains the most sustainable in the long run. So your breakdown of habits may look something like this:

» **Week 1:** I'll run for 30 minutes on Tuesday morning before work. I'll place my running gear and trainers next to my bed the night before (trigger).

» **Week 4:** I'll run for 30 minutes on Tuesday and Thursday mornings before work. I'll place my running gear and trainers next to my bed the night before (trigger).

» **Week 9:** I'll run for 30 minutes on Tuesday, Wednesday, and Thursday mornings before work. I'll place my running gear and trainers next to my bed the night before (trigger). After my shower (trigger), I'll have a balanced breakfast to refuel.

» **Week 16:** I'll run for 30 minutes on Monday, Tuesday, Wednesday, and Thursday mornings before work. I'll place my running gear and trainers next to my bed the night before (trigger). After my shower (trigger), I'll have a balanced breakfast to refuel.

» **Week 24:** I'll run for 30 minutes on Monday, Tuesday, Wednesday, and Thursday mornings before work. I'll place my running gear and trainers next to my bed the night before (trigger). After my shower (trigger), I'll have a balanced breakfast to refuel. While I make breakfast (trigger), I'll also pack a homemade lunch to bring to work.

» **Week 36:** I'll run for 30 minutes on Monday, Tuesday, Wednesday, Thursday, and Friday mornings before work. I'll place my running gear and trainers next to my bed the night before (trigger). After my shower (trigger), I'll have a balanced breakfast to refuel. While I make breakfast (trigger), I'll also pack a homemade lunch to bring to work.

Do you see what happens? Not only are you able to slowly become accustomed to your new habit, allowing yourself time to optimise and improve it, but you also develop both secondary healthy habits. This type of introduced routine is known as a keystone habit.

According to Charles Duhigg (2014), author of *The Power of Habit: Why We Do What We Do in Life and Business*, a keystone habit is one that has a positive influence on other aspects of your life and creates a chain reaction of positive habits that infiltrate your everyday routine. In this example, by increasing your daily exercise, you subconsciously improved your breakfast habits. This may be a result of increased hunger from increased energy expenditure and your prioritisation of health, but the development of one healthy habit has influenced you to make a second healthy habit, and even a third. Due to your increase in exercise, you may also feel less stressed, consume more fluids, improve your sleep, and increase your productivity at work. While you may not see these results right away, just remember that small positive changes can snowball into bigger lifestyle shifts.

Here's another example of how gratitude can act as a keystone habit:

**daily gratitude ➜ increased positivity ➜ increased self-compassion ➜ increased body satisfaction ➜ increased self-esteem and confidence ➜ improved relationships**

According to James Clear, the idea of making daily micro-improvements can be referred to as 'the power of tiny gains' (Duhigg 2014). This theory states that by improving yourself or your habits (remember, we're the sum of our habits), you can improve by 37.78 percent a year.

So remember, change doesn't happen overnight. Developing small, positive habits can help lead to bigger shifts over time. Start small so your habit becomes your routine, which results in decisions made on autopilot. Remember, it starts with your trigger.

To help you kick-start some of your healthy habits, here's an activity.* Create a chart similar to the following for at least 10 weeks. Fill it out to see if you've kept up with your positive habits so that they'll become routine.

| Cue: | | | | | | |
|---|---|---|---|---|---|---|
| Motivation: | | | | | | |
| Response: | | | | | | |
| Reward: | | | | | | |
| Week 1 | | | | | | |
| Monday | Tuesday | Wednesday | Thursday | Friday | Saturday | Sunday |
| | | | | | | |

Done on more than 5 days, Y/N?

How automatic does it feel (scale of 1-10)?

| Week 2 | | | | | | |
|---|---|---|---|---|---|---|
| Monday | Tuesday | Wednesday | Thursday | Friday | Saturday | Sunday |
| | | | | | | |

Done on more than 5 days, Y/N?

How automatic does it feel (scale of 1-10)?

*Adapted from Gardner, Lally, and Wardle 2012.

# How to Get Confident
# in the Kitchen

Feeling confident in the kitchen can be one of the most important steps towards making healthy and lasting changes. We completely understand that not everyone enjoys cooking or spending time in the kitchen. But not to worry—we have some helpful tips to inspire you and leave you feeling optimistic.

We'll teach you some helpful strategies and educate you on the essentials of what you need to know to feel confident in the kitchen.

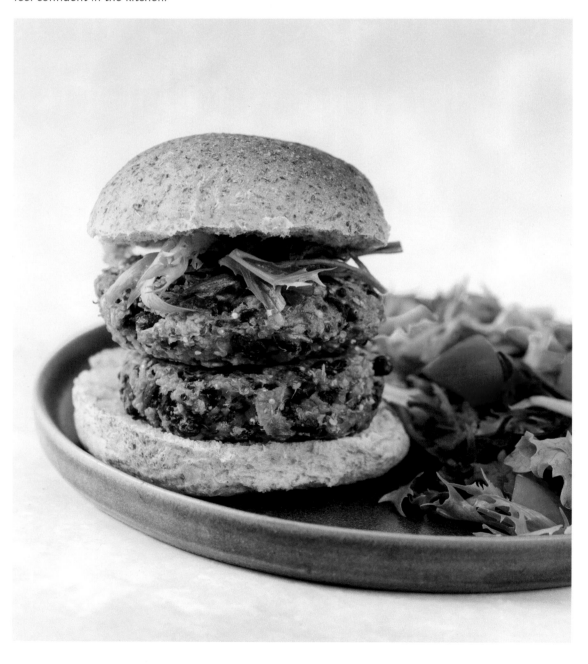

# How to Make a Meal Plan

If you've listened to our podcast, you might remember—from one of our very first episodes—our discussion about meal plans. In our experience, meal plans are great for anyone who's busy, has to cook around multiple preferences or dietary restrictions, or wants to save a bit of money. Now, we know everyone will approach this differently, especially depending on the number of people you're cooking for. But we like to take the time over the weekend to map out our meals for the following week.

These are the things to consider:

» how many people you're cooking for

» how many meals you need to prepare for—is it just dinners, or do you also need lunches?

» preferences

» diversity

» availability and offers—we highly recommend you check online for deals and offers at your local supermarket to help save money

» any freezer items you can incorporate—for example, previously batch-cooked foods you froze

If you need to cook for lunches and dinners both, our biggest tips include setting aside some time for batch cooking or making extra portions at dinner, to take with you the next day.

Now, when it comes to choosing what foods to make, you want to consider how you can use leftover ingredients in future meals. This will help eliminate food waste and also save you money. For example, if you buy a bunch of mushrooms and use only half of them in a recipe—say, our Sweet-Potato Hash-Brown Frittata —finding another recipe to utilise the remaining of the mushrooms is essential.

While we don't believe in providing you with a meal plan to try, because we know everyone is different with regard to their current place in their health journey, preferences, and more, we do want to show you an example.

Here's how we make our weekly meal plans and the things we consider:

» two dinners every night and five lunches

» one fish meal per week

» differing food preferences

» using the same ingredients to make different meals, to minimise food waste

Here's what a sample week might look like:

| Sample Week Meal Plan | | | | | |
|---|---|---|---|---|---|
| | Monday | Tuesday | Wednesday | Thursday | Friday |
| Bari's lunch | leftovers from the previous night's dinner | leftover veggie stir-fry with added edamame cashews, and brown rice | leftover coconut dahl | leftover coconut dahl | veggie burger over spinach salad and chickpeas |
| Bari's dinner | veggie stir-fry with salmon and brown rice | coconut dahl | gnocchi, ratatouille with leftover veg, and chickpeas | veggie burger, spinach salad, roasted carrots, and garlic bread | breakfast for dinner: avocado toast with scrambled eggs, halloumi, and rocket (arugula) |
| Mark's dinner | veggie stir-fry with salmon and brown rice | coconut dahl and added chicken thighs | gnocchi, spinach, and spicy sausages | spicy Asian chicken thighs, roasted carrots, spinach salad, and garlic bread | breakfast for dinner: avocado toast with scrambled eggs, halloumi, leftover sausages, and rocket |

| | Monday | Tuesday | Wednesday | Thursday | Friday |
|---|---|---|---|---|---|
| Sophie's lunch | courgette (zucchini) fritters | leftover veggie quinoa bake | leftover courgette (zucchini) fritters | leftover veggie pasta | falafel wraps |
| Sophie's dinner | veggie quinoa bake | tomato and lentil soup with bread | veggie pasta | tofu teriyaki stir-fry with brown rice and veg | homemade nachos |
| Ash's dinner | cod, mash, and veg | Chicken-and-veg-soup with bread | veggie pasta | chicken teriyaki stir-fry with brown rice and veg | homemade nachos |

Obviously, not everyone has such complicated situations, and if you're cooking for another person, hopefully you can both enjoy the same meal. But this shows how to add some structure to make things easier and more affordable.

Why aren't we writing a sample menu? We don't believe in designing meal plans for others.

As nutrition professionals, we both work with private clients. But we don't give out specific meal plans, because—as mentioned at the start of the book—everyone should be entitled to eat how they see fit, depending on their own individual needs and desires. This may lead you to question how we work with clients. We believe in giving individuals guidance and helping them to rely on their own body in order to determine their diet.

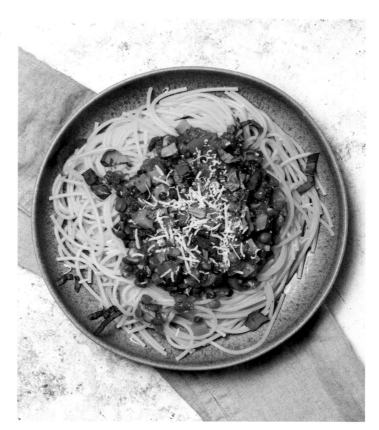

## WHY STRUCTURE IS IMPORTANT

Now, you may be thinking that the structure of a meal plan seems rigid or counterintuitive to our philosophy of listening to your body and cravings. And while that may be true to an extent, creating a rough idea of what you're going to cook for the week is also a helpful tool when it comes to getting organised and planning your weekly food shop. In an ideal world, you'd ask yourself, What do I want to eat tonight? You'd then pop to the shop, pick up your ingredients, and cook a lovely meal. But things such as work, commutes, financial caution, limited time, and a lack of motivation make that difficult. At the end of the day, this book is all about providing you with practical and realistic recommendations to help you make positive and healthy choices, and for some, including us, that means writing a meal plan for the week ahead.

For most, writing down the meals you plan to make is a great way to stay organised and accountable. You might use this as an opportunity to try new recipes or new ingredients. Or if you're a novice home cook, you can use this as a helpful strategy to practise new cooking techniques. Also, if you're trying to build new healthy habits, such as bringing a packed lunch to work every day, making a meal plan may be the strategy you need to help you achieve your goal.

The key to having a meal plan for the week is allowing for flexibility. If you feel that writing down your future food promotes rigid, restrictive, or obsessive behaviours, then this isn't for you. Just remember, everyone is on a different journey towards health and happiness, and adapting your strategies to suit your needs is the most important approach. If you feel like a meal plan can provide you with the structure and organisation you need, that's brilliant. We personally find a meal plan to be helpful in our busy and hectic lives. But we both know that the plan we write at the start of the week isn't written in stone. Scrapping the intended plan and going out for dinner, ordering a takeaway, swapping around meals, or simply having beans on toast for a quick, no-cook meal is absolutely OK. There's no shame in deviating from the plan, especially because the day's events can be unpredictable.

But if you're trying to build healthy habits, such as increasing your vegetable intake, trying new foods, or cooking from scratch, writing a meal plan can be a positive strategy.

# Eating Seasonally

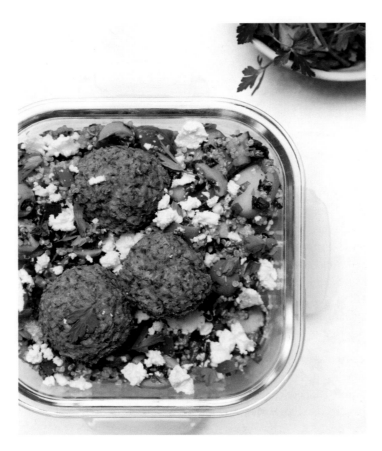

Seasonal eating involves eating foods according to them being harvested at a specific time of year, at which point they're at their peak with regard to flavour and quality. Eating foods that are in season can also help reduce greenhouse-gas emissions, therefore, we should all aim to make an effort to be mindful of food choices at different times of the year. We know what you're thinking: something else to consider?! But don't worry, we're here to make it a little easier, and we've put together an easy-read chart you can refer to when needed.

| Seasonal Foods (UK) | | | |
|---|---|---|---|
| January | February | March | April |
| **Fruits** | **Fruits** | **Fruits** | **Fruits** |
| apples, pears | apples, pears | rhubarb | rhubarb |
| **Veggies** | **Veggies** | **Veggies** | **Veggies** |
| beetroot, brussels sprouts, cabbage, carrots, chicory, jerusalem artichokes, kale, leeks, mushrooms, onions, parsnips, spring greens, spring onions, squash, swede, turnips | beetroot, brussels sprouts, cabbage, carrots, celeriac, chicory, jerusalem artichokes, kale, leeks, mushrooms, onions, parsnips, purple-sprouting broccoli, spring greens, spring onions, squash, swede | artichokes, beetroot, cabbage, carrots, chicory, cucumbers, leeks, parsnips, purple-sprouting broccoli, radishes, sorrel, spring greens, spring onions, watercress | artichokes, beetroot, cabbage, carrots, chicory, kale, morel mushrooms, new potatoes, parsnips, radishes, rocket, sorrel, spinach, spring greens, spring onions, watercress |
| May | June | July | August |
| **Fruits** | **Fruits** | **Fruits** | **Fruits** |
| elderflowers, rhubarb, strawberries | black currants, cherries, elderflowers, gooseberries, raspberries, red currants, rhubarb, strawberries, tayberries | blackberries, black currants, blueberries, cherries, gooseberries, loganberries, raspberries, red currants, rhubarb, strawberries | blackberries, black currants, cherries, damsons, greengagesl mange-tout oganberries, plums, raspberries, red currants, rhubarb, strawberries |
| **Veggies** | **Veggies** | **Veggies** | **Veggies** |
| artichokes, asparagus, aubergine, beetroot, chicory, chillies, lettuce, marrow, new potatoes, peas, peppers, radishes, rocket, samphire, sorrel, spinach, spring greens, spring onions, watercress | asparagus, aubergine, beetroot, broad beans, broccoli, cauliflower, chicory, chillies, courgettes, cucumber | aubergine, beetroot, broad beans, broccoli, carrots, cauliflower, chicory, chillies, courgette, cucumbers, greengages, fennel, french beans, garlic, kohlrabi, new potatoes, onions, peas, potatoes, radishes, rocket, runner beans, samphire, sorrel, spring greens, spring onions, summer squash, swiss chard, tomatoes, turnips, watercress | aubergine, beetroot, broad beans, broccoli, carrots, cauliflower, chicory, chillies, courgette, cucumbers, fennel, french beans, garlic, greengages, kohlrabi, leeks, lettuce, mange-touts, marrow, mushrooms, parsnips, peas, peppers, potatoes, pumpkin, radishes, rocket, runner beans, samphire, sorrel, spring greens, spring onions, summer squash, sweetcorn, swiss chard, tomatoes, watercress |

| September | October | November | December |
|---|---|---|---|
| **Fruits** | **Fruits** | **Fruits** | **Fruits** |
| blackberries, damsons pears, plums, raspberries, rhubarb, strawberries | apples, blackberries, elderberries, pears | apples, cranberries, elderberries | apples, cranberries, pears |
| **Veggies** | **Veggies** | **Veggies** | **Veggies** |
| aubergine, beetroot, broccoli, brussels sprouts, butternut squash, carrots, cauliflower, celery, chicory, chillies, courgette, cucumbers, garlic, kale, kohlrabi, leeks, lettuce, mange-touts, marrow, onions, parsnips, peas, peppers, potatoes, pumpkin, radishes, rocket, runner beans, samphire, sorrel, spinach, spring greens, spring onions, summer squash, sweet corn, swiss chard, tomatoes, turnips, watercress, wild mushrooms | aubergine, beetroot, broccoli, brussels sprouts, butternut squash, carrots, cauliflower, celeriac, celery, chestnut mushrooms chicory, chillies, courgette, cucumbers, kale, leeks, lettuce, marrow, onions, parsnips, peas, potatoes, pumpkin, radishes, rocket, runner beans, spinach, spring greens, spring onions, summer squash, swede, sweet corn, swiss chard, tomatoes, turnips, watercress, wild mushrooms, winter squash | beetroot, brussels sprouts, butternut squash, cabbage, carrots, cauliflower, celeriac, celery, chestnuts, chicory, jerusalem artichokes, kale, leeks, onions, parsnips, potatoes, pumpkin, swede, swiss chard, turnips, watercress, wild mushrooms, winter squash | beetroot, brussels sprouts, carrots, celeriac, celery, chestnuts, chicory, jerusalem artichokes, kale, leeks, mushrooms, onions, parsnips, potatoes, pumpkin, red cabbage, swede, swiss chard, turnips, watercress, winter squash |

You'll likely notice that foods that are in season have extra flavour and enhanced textures and are juicier. The best example is strawberries: you can't beat a bunch of juicy strawberries in the summer months—they taste so much better.

*Top Tip*

**Buy frozen berries. They're cheaper and are picked and frozen at their peak, so they contain the same (if not more) nutrients.**

# Eating Sustainably

## WHAT DOES IT MEAN TO EAT SUSTAINABLY?

A sustainable diet is commonly associated with having a positive impact on the environment. Additionally, there's emerging research indicating it's a healthful way in which we can eat too, therefore benefiting the environment and perhaps encouraging healthy eating behaviours as well. Sustainable eating puts emphasis on eating more plant foods, which is likely to result in increased fibre intake (which we know is beneficial to our health). In fact, vegan and vegetarian diets have been noted to have significant reduction in land use and greenhouse-gas emissions (Willett et al. 2019).

According to the World Health Organization (2018), food production accounts for 20–30 percent of global greenhouse-gas emissions.

We don't believe you need to place labels on the way in which you choose to eat, but this research simply demonstrates that a diet focused on plant-based foods can really can have a positive impact on the world around us. Plant-based eaters generally include a variety of fruits, veg, whole grains, nuts, and legumes in their diet.

## HOW DO WE EAT SUSTAINABLY?

If making a conscious effort to eat more sustainably is a new concept for you, we advise you take it one step at a time. Helping to look after our environment via food intake isn't supposed to feel restrictive, and it's a matter of making a few small changes to enable you to feel like you're doing something good for the planet. Making a huge change all of sudden may cause feelings of chaos and do more harm than good with regard to your eating patterns. If you'd like to decrease the amount of meat you're eating, simply start by dedicating one to two days a week to plant products. A lot of people like the term *meatless Monday* as it's an easy way to remember your plant-food day. You can also try alternating your meals—if you're used to having meat as your main protein source at each meal, start experimenting with some plant proteins too.

*Top Tip*

**If you're not used to plant-protein sources, try seasoning them, for extra flavour.**

Before we dive in and share some stats, know that we're simply providing you with knowledge so you can make informed decisions. This isn't a section where we tell you how much of what foods you should be eating, but we believe sustainability is an important part of living life healthfully.

## MEAT

Meat has a pretty high environmental impact, and as a country, we're eating too much of it. Quality meat products can be very nutritious and are particularly good sources of complete proteins. But we know from existing research that excessive red-meat consumption may increase one's risk of certain diseases, such as heart disease. Lowering your meat consumption isn't only beneficial for the environment but can also encourage you to add more variety to your diet, helping to diversify your gut microbiome, thus contributing to overall well-being.

## FISH

Unfortunately, a lot of fish stocks are becoming depleted due to overfishing, thus, it's having a detrimental effect on the environment. You can be mindful when purchasing fish and check (on the label) whether or not it was sustainably sourced. Fatty fish, such as salmon and mackerel, are good sources of omega-3s, which are essential and therefore nutritious additions to one's diet. But there are plenty of plant-based sources and alternate ways you can make sure you're getting adequate amounts of omega-3 should you not consume fatty fish. (See the 'Nutrition Basics' chapter earlier in the book.)

## DAIRY

Dairy is another food group that's considered to have a relatively high impact on the environment, but it's important to consider the nutritional value of products such as milk and yoghurt. Whilst being affordable, they're also a primary source of essential vitamins and minerals such as vitamin D, calcium, phosphorus, and iodine. But, unlike 20 years ago, we now have access to a variety of alternative dairy products that are fortified with nutrients, such as vitamin D, calcium, vitamin B12 (which is difficult to get enough of on a vegan diet), and phosphorus—and some with iodine too. If you're opting for plant-based milk and yoghurt to replace dairy, fortification is important, so always check the label.

## FRUITS AND VEG

Fruits and veggies have relatively low impact on the environment, however, according to Public Health England (2018), only 31 percent of adults, 32 percent of people 65–74 years old, and 8 percent of teenagers meet the 5 A Day recommendation for fruit and vegetables. Fruits and veg are an extremely nutritious part of our diet. We can all be mindful when buying these types of foods and think about the seasons and buy organic when we can. There's a misconception that *organic* means healthier, but in the UK, there's limited research to say this is the case. Nevertheless, buying organic does work in our environment's favour. Fruits and veggies that are farmed organically conserve water, reduce soil erosion, and use less energy. You don't *have* to buy organic, since we're aware that this often comes with added expense, but it's good to know the facts to make an informed choice.

## PREPACKAGED FOODS

Although we're making progress with regard to reducing the amount of packaging we use in supermarkets, we still have a long way to go. Reducing the amount of products you buy that contain excess packaging can really have an impact in the long run. Use your own eco-friendly bags to pick up fresh produce, take your own shopping bags, and even go as far as making your own snacks.

## WHAT ELSE CAN WE DO?

There are small steps you can begin to include in your lifestyle to help contribute to looking after our environment, and the following tips are a great place to start.

## PLAN YOUR MEALS AND MAKE A SHOPPING LIST

You don't need to be super strict with regard to knowing exactly what you're going to eat each day, but it's helpful to plan what meals you can curate out of the ingredients you buy. If you walk into the supermarket and pick foods at random, they may end up going to waste. Additionally, we've both been caught by the two-for-one deals—ask yourself if you're genuinely going to finish each food before it expires or if you're just being lured in by the sale price. If you live alone, you may find it more strategic to do a food shop twice a week, since a lot of fresh foods have a short shelf life. For more help planning meals and budgeting to reduce food waste, see page 101.

## TRY MEATLESS DAYS

As you may have gathered from this section you don't have to cut meat out altogether, but reducing meat intake will have a positive impact on the environment. Try switching out your animal proteins for plant proteins a few days of the week, or maybe halve your usual meat portion and top up with a plant alternative too. For example, you could use half mincemeat and half lentils.

## SWITCH IT UP

It's easy to fall into the food-trend traps. We're both guilty of this. But something we learned through our personal research, as well as shared on an episode on the *Forking Wellness* podcast, is how food trends can put undue burdens and pressures on farmers and our natural resources.

### The Domino Effect of Food Trends

#### Avocado

Did you know that avocados are referred to as 'green gold'? A 2019 report written by Christian Wagner states that the exportation of avocados from Mexico was worth $2.4 billion in 2018. While this is incredible for the Mexican economy and farmers, record-breaking sales have attracted the likes of organised crime, specifically Mexican cartels. According to Wagner (2019), organised crime operations are taking advantage of the mass exportation of avocados, specifically to smuggle contraband and fighting over everything from avocado-producing regions to trade routes.

While we're not telling you to skip your avocado toast, you may want to switch it up and try other toppings, such as hummus or mashed green peas.

#### Quinoa

Before you found quinoa (pronounced KEEN-waa) in your local Whole Foods Market, quinoa was a major food staple in places like Bolivia and Peru. The demand for this nutritious grain sent the price sky-high, eventually making it so expensive even the farmers could no longer afford it. Essentially, the Western demand for this trendy yet delicious food displaced it from the diet of the poor farmers, causing them to rely on cheaper, more-processed food (Yu 2019).

# Enjoy Leftovers

Not only are leftovers perfect for meal prepping, but they also help to reduce food waste. You can create lunch boxes to take to work, use up veggies to make a soup, blend fruits to make a smoothie, or even freeze certain foods and meals to preserve them.

## STOCK UP ON REUSABLE GOODS

Don't throw away your plastic—wash it out and use it again. Don't go to a coffee shop without your eco-friendly coffee cup. Don't use plastic straws; try a bamboo or metal one and reuse it. Refill your water bottle. All these things make a difference, so encourage your friends to do the same.

You don't need to feel overwhelmed by this information and start making extreme changes. We believe it's more sustainable to make small changes over time, and if you'd like more guidance on sustainable eating, you can visit the BDA website and find their One Blue Dot toolkit (BDA 2019).

# For Fussy Eaters

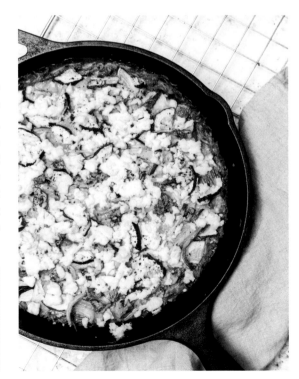

If you're a parent, you might be thinking, But my child is so fussy, or you might even be the fussy one. We know that diversity in the diet is beneficial, but this can be tricky if your taste buds aren't keen on a variety of foods. You may have noticed that in some of the chapters, we like to share 'top tips' that you can take away from a specific topic to (hopefully) help you make small and easy yet effective changes. So here are our top tips for fussy eaters.

A 2017 study reveals that 50 percent of parents described their children as fussy eaters (Walton et al. 2017).

## INTRODUCE YOURSELF (OR YOUR CHILD) TO NEW FOODS AND GET CREATIVE

If you don't try, you'll never know, but don't stop there. If you don't like boiled vegetables, for example, try roasting them in the oven, seasoned with olive oil. Trust us, they taste completely different. You might not like raw onion, but you might love it chopped up and flavoured in a stew. You might not like cold quinoa in a salad, but you might like it hot and served with roasted veg and salmon. See where we're going with this? Our favourite thing to do is make a veggie burger (see our recipe index), because you can't always tell how much diversity you're eating otherwise, and as long as you get the flavours right, you're onto a winner.

## TRY MINDFUL EATING

Mindful eating (although not for everyone) can really enhance your eating experience. We want everyone to find eating enjoyable, and if you rush your food down, you can't always identify whether or not it was a pleasant experience.

## GET IN THE KITCHEN AND START COOKING

You don't need to be a professional chef or talented cook to produce delicious foods. Taking time to cook from scratch can enhance the whole eating experience and help you get to know how you enjoy having your meals cooked. Although we're aware it's not possible to set aside time to do this every day, you can prioritise time a few days a week to cook up a meal, then sit and enjoy what you've made.

## REMEMBER THAT YOU'RE IN CHARGE OF YOUR OWN BODY

You don't have to enjoy all foods. You can like and dislike as many foods as you want to as long as you're happy and feel like you're getting a large enough variety of nutrients. Don't let anyone judge your food choices—just find what works for you.

We hope that by now you feel confident in the fact that you get to be in charge of your own body and you're the one person who'll understand your body more than anyone. You just have to trust yourself.

# Kitchen Staples

## HERBS AND SPICES

Let's touch on the wonderful world of herbs and spices—such small ingredients that can quite literally transform our food and cooking. Aside from the fact that they carry so much flavour, they have the added bonus of nutritional value. We've highlighted a few herbs and spices in particular that (we think) are wonderful to cook with, and we have some supporting evidence with regard to their added nutritional benefit.

### Cinnamon

The following things are true of cinnamon:

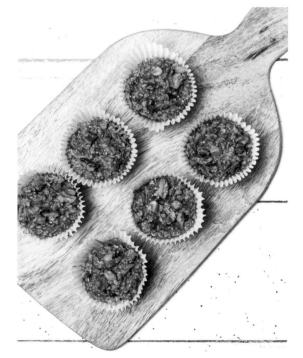

» It's a versatile spice that can enhance most baked goods. In addition to having its sweet, aromatic flavour, cinnamon has also been suggested to contain antioxidant properties that may help fight inflammation (El-Baroty et al. 2010; Shan et al. 2005).

» There's also a small amount of supporting research to indicate that this spice may help lower blood-sugar levels and improve insulin sensitivity (Qin, Panickar, and Anderson 2010).

» Specific studies have actually shown that cinnamon may lower fasting blood sugars in patients with diabetes (Pham, Kourlas, and Pham 2007).

» A typical serving size is anything from ½ to 2 tsp.

We love cinnamon in our porridge bowls, pancakes, breads, and cookies or biscuits.

### Peppermint

Peppermint has been linked to helping with the management of pain, IBS, relaxing muscles, and digestive symptoms, such as bloating (Khanna, MacDonald, and Levesque 2014; Ford et al. 2008).

There's some research to suggest that peppermint may help to reduce feelings of nausea, however, more studies are needed to confirm this, as it may be due to the techniques at which the peppermint is administered, as opposed to the peppermint itself (Anderson and Gross 2004).

We find peppermint tea enjoyable towards the end of the day as it contains no caffeine, but you can also add it to baked goods—think: mint chocolate cookies!

### Ginger

Another spice that sits at the top of our favourites list—ginger. Like peppermint, ginger may also be linked to possibly managing pain and may contain anti-inflammatory properties (Black et al. 2010). Ginger is often highlighted for its ability to settle the stomach and fight nausea. Studies have suggested that just one gram of ginger can have a positive effect with regard to reducing nausea caused by morning sickness, sea sickness, and even chemotherapy (Ernst and Pittler 2000).

### Turmeric

Probably the spice with the most hype around it and, of course, the foundation of a golden-milk latte is turmeric. What's important to remember is that one single addition to your diet is unlikely to work a miracle, but if you genuinely like the taste of the spice, there's some supporting research to say it may provide some health benefits. Curcumin is the compound in turmeric that gives that potent colour and is actually why it's thought to have some medicinal properties (Nagpal and Sood 2013). Curcumin is an antioxidant, and we know from research that antioxidants help reduce oxidative damage, which is thought to be a driving factor in terms of how quickly we age (Menon and Sudheer 2007; Barclay et al. 2000).

We suggest spicing up your favourite curry with some turmeric spice.

Other studies suggest that this potent spice may help improve cognitive function and help manage arthritis (Mishra and Palanivelu 2008; Chandran and Goel 2012).

Although there's some promising research, we'd have to be consuming significant amounts of turmeric to feel the effects, and there are plenty of other foods we can get a variety of antioxidants from.

### Garlic

Historically, garlic has been used for its perceived health benefits (Rivlin 2001). The theory is that garlic can help fight off minor illnesses such as coughs and colds, and there's some evidence to support this as garlic may increase the body's production of natural killer cells (Josling 2001; Nantz et al. 2012).

There are also studies that demonstrate a positive link between including garlic in one's diet and maintaining a healthy heart. Research suggests that garlic may help reduce high cholesterol and high blood pressure (Sobenin et al. 2008; Sutherland et al. 2009).

You can use garlic in any of your savoury dishes and buy it frozen from supermarkets so it lasts longer and is easy to use.

Although there's evidence to support medicinal properties in herbs and spices, hopefully you know by now that there's no miracle food, so please don't rely on adding these ingredients to food in order to improve certain health conditions. We're simply highlighting that, as well as adding flavour to food, these ingredients carry nutritional value too.

## FRUITS AND VEGGIES

Fruits and veggies always brighten up a dish, and we know from extensive research that they're an essential part of a well-balanced diet, providing us with a whole variety of vitamins and minerals (micronutrients) that promote good health. The more colour, the more nutrients, so it's important to add as much as you see fit to your overall diet. Although we've all heard of the recommended 5 A Day, there's emerging research that tells us that eating more than five servings (in fact, research suggests it should be around 10) can be really beneficial (NHS 2017).

We understand that not everyone has the means to buy an abundance of different fruits and veggies all the time, and we also want everyone to be mindful of limiting food waste, too, so even if you can afford as much as you like, we certainly don't want it going to waste. So here are three different ways you can buy what you need to suit your lifestyle.

**Fresh**

Try and be realistic when thinking about fresh-food consumption. We know that fresh berries, for example, tend to lose their freshness after a few days and become less appealing to eat. So if you live on your own or think that a punnet of berries won't be finished within a few days, it may be more practical to opt for frozen (which are cheaper too). Same with veg. We like to freeze bags of spinach because a bag tends to go bad after three or four days. Note that while it's very unlikely you'll get ill from eating fruits and veg past their use-by dates, we all know that when it doesn't look as fresh as when we brought it we may be less likely to eat it and more likely to bin it. Broccoli is one we like to buy fresh, and we go through it pretty quickly. Decide what's realistic for you—you can also refer to the seasonal-eating section for reference.

**Frozen**

Buying frozen is a real money saver—and you can also rest knowing that fruits and vegetables are picked at their peak and frozen almost instantly, so there's no compromising with regard to nutritional value. Bags of peas and of sweet corn are great additions to your freezer as they're cheap and a source of fibre and micronutrients. They can easily be added to pastas, stews, fritters, and casseroles. Berries, bananas, avocados, chunks of mango, and pineapple are also fab to stick in the freezer.

### Tinned

Tinned foods like beans, lentils, chickpeas, tomatoes, and fruits all count towards your fruit and veg intake for the day. They're very cheap, often costing around 40p–90p per can. Again, these foods can easily be added to a variety of dishes and can help you save money too. They often have a long shelf life, so it doesn't matter if you leave them sitting in your cupboard until you fancy eating them.

### Microwaveable Packs

Now, these really are cupboard staples. They make cooking main meals so much quicker and easier. A few years ago, a pack of microwaveable grains was around £2.50, but now supermarkets have released their own brands, and you can buy yourself a pack that serves two for as little as 65p. This includes rice, freekeh, lentils, quinoa, and other mixed grains. They make for a great lunch-box base or can be quickly heated to add to your main meal when you don't have time to cook. They're also a convenient way to increase your fibre intake and contain other essential nutrients.

### Oils

There are a lot of misconceptions with regard to what oils are best to cook with, and a lot of people associate oils with being unhealthy. No type of oil is bad for us; we just need to consider how, how much, and how often we're using it. Oils can be used in so many different ways and can really enhance your cooking experience and the overall taste of a meal. Additionally, oils provide us with important nutrients and may aid the absorption of micronutrients, however, nutrients might become compromised, depending on how you use the oils. So let's break it down.

Consider these things when using oils:

» the smoke point

» how you're using them (e.g. cooking, salad dressing)

» cost

» taste

» environmental impact

**Extra-Virgin Olive Oil:** This may be one of the most popular cooking oils, and it's also one of the most researched oils. Studies show that EVOO is rich in antioxidants, contains healthy fats that help support good heart health, and has been linked to reduced risk of cancer and cardiovascular disease (Trichopoulou et al. 2000; Owen et al. 2004; Owen et al. 2000).

For a more unprocessed and less refined option, you may want to opt for EVOO. But it's important to be aware of the smoke points of cooking oils. *Smoke point* refers to the temperature in which an oil starts to burn and release potentially damaging free radicals. If you're using an oil for frying or roasting, you ideally need to be using one with a high smoke point. EVOO has a smoke point of around 191°C (375°F), which means that in order to reap the perceived health benefits it's best used as a dressing or dip and not heated. You can use regular olive oil (which contains a lot of the same health benefits) for frying, sautéing, grilling, and similar high-heat preparation method as olive oil has a higher smoke point of around 243°C (470°F).

**Coconut Oil:** Coconut oil has gained increased interest over the years and, like most oils, you can find refined and unrefined (also called *virgin*) versions of it. Both refined and unrefined coconut oil have smoke points of 232°C (450°F) and 177°C (350°F), respectively. Coconut oil can make for a really delicious cooking oil, particularly when it comes to making Thai recipes, curries, and sweet baked recipes. It's also popular as an oil in raw desserts. In the last few years, there's been a fair amount of controversy regarding coconut oil, some labelling it a superfood and some referring to it as a bad oil. It really doesn't fall into either of those dramatic categories and, if used in appropriate quantities (around one to two tsp per serving), can be part of a healthy balanced diet. Coconut oil is made up of approximately 90 percent saturated fat, so we suggest you be mindful of your overall consumption.

**Rapeseed Oil:** Rapeseed oil (canola oil) is another popular oil to cook with. It's a vegetable oil that's used in a lot of food products, and you'll likely see this ingredient often on food labels. It's inexpensive and has a neutral taste. This is another oil that's ideal for cooking as it has a high smoke point of 204°C (400°F). But traditional rapeseed oil is often highly processed; therefore, we recommend opting for cold-pressed when you can and drizzling it on salads—yum!

**Sesame Oil:** A source of essential fats and antioxidants, sesame oil makes for a versatile cooking oil, with a smoke point of around 204°C (400°F) and is best stored in the fridge. Again, if you can, opt for the unprocessed version—cold-pressed sesame oil. We love it lightly drizzled at the end of a stir-fry.

**Avocado Oil:** Avocado oil (like avocados) is a good source of monounsaturated fats and makes for an excellent cooking oil due to the fact that it has a very high smoke point—270°C (520°F) for refined and around 250C (480°F) for unrefined. But this oil is one of the more expensive ones on the shelf and isn't very sustainable, so this probably isn't your everyday oil.

For day-to-day cooking, rapeseed and light olive oil are ideal options, and you can switch it up with other oils depending on what flavours you desire for specific dishes.

**Storing Oils:** Oils need to be kept away from direct sunlight as they're sensitive to heat and light, so store them in a dark, cool, dry place and always make sure the cap is on nice and tight once used. If the oil smells 'off', you may need to replace it.

(American Heart Association 2018)

# Cheesy Bean and Quinoa Bake

Here's why it's great:

» cheap

» nutritious

» source of complete protein

» easy to make

» ideal for lunch boxes

» vegan option

**Yield:** 3 to 4 servings

**Cook time:** 35-45 minutes

## Ingredients

2-3 tbsp olive oil

1 tsp paprika

1 medium onion, chopped (We recommend buying prechopped packs that can be kept in the freezer.)

1 (400 g or 15 oz.) tin tomatoes

2 (400 g or 15 oz.) tins mixed beans, drained

1 tin jackfruit 400 g or 15 oz.) (optional)

170 g (1 cup) quinoa

100 mL water

3 tbsp tomato puree

1 tbsp nutritional yeast (optional)

Salt and cracked black pepper to taste

60 g grated cheddar or vegan cheese (optional)

## Method

1. Preheat the oven to 180°C (350°F).

2. Heat the olive oil, paprika, and onions in a pan over medium-high heat.

3. Once the onions start to brown, add the tinned tomatoes, beans, jackfruit, quinoa, and water and lower the heat down to medium-low so it can simmer for 10 to 15 minutes.

4. Add the tomato puree, nutritional yeast, salt, and pepper and stir until the quinoa is cooked, usually about 10 minutes.

5. Transfer to an oven-safe dish and sprinkle the grated cheese on top.

6. Bake in the oven for 15–20 minutes, until the cheese is melted and slightly crispy. Enjoy!

# Conclusion

The statements following this paragraph are examples of wellness—some might apply to you, and some might not; but, hopefully, after reading our approach, you have a much better idea of what *healthy* means to you. If you live a busy life, convenience might be a priority—this means being prepared, meal prepping, and making sure you have those go-to, easy-to-cook kitchen staples. You might be trying to heal your relationship with food, so prioritising intuitive eating may be important. Or you may simply be trying to increase your fruit and veg intake. Everyone will have a different goal or preference with regard to how he or she wants to eat and live life. We hope this book has given you the tools you need to do that. You don't have to apply every section of the book to your lifestyle. Instead, pick and choose what's relevant and important to you.

**Wellness is . . .**

- » eating your vegetables
- » having a cookie
- » taking a 20-minute walk each day
- » talking to your best friend every week
- » having three meals a day
- » having six meals a day
- » drinking 2 L of water
- » reading your favourite book
- » laughing with your kids
- » drinking wine with friends
- » eating a box of chocolates on movie night
- » experimenting with new recipes
- » prepping lunch boxes
- » accepting your body
- » loving your body
- » choosing to eat for taste, not health
- » nourishing your mind
- » skipping your workout
- » challenging yourself to a new workout
- » building healthy habits
- » honouring your cravings
- » having a green smoothie
- » practising self-care
- » accidently falling asleep with your makeup on
- » snoozing your alarm clock
- » being productive
- » mindfully eating
- » eating for comfort
- » having no regrets
- » being unapologetically you

So—what the fork is wellness?
In a world where everything is wellness, nothing is wellness.
Prioritise yourself, your happiness, and your health without sacrifice and call it whatever the fork you want.

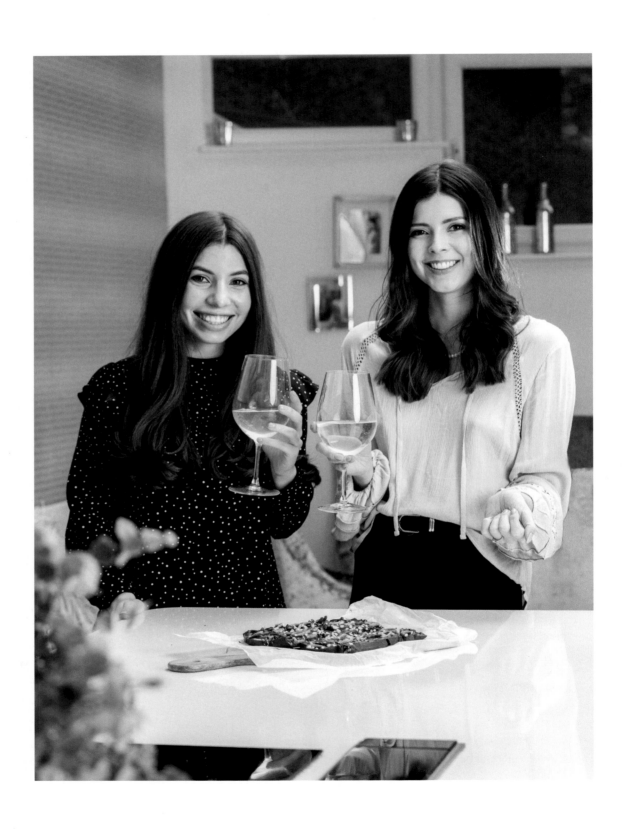

# Recipes

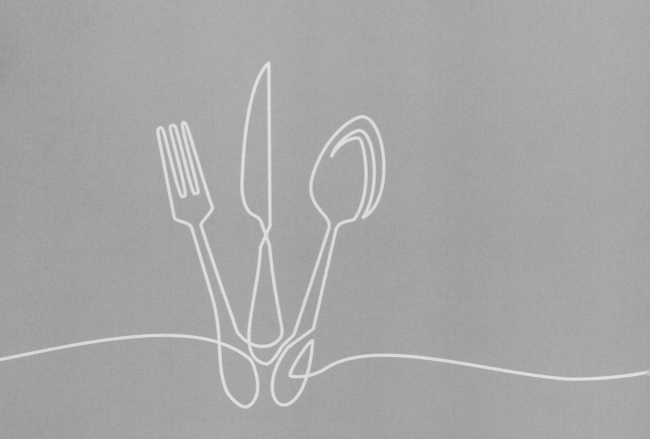

# Breakfast

In our eyes, breakfast is the best part of the morning. We've developed a variety of recipes that will enhance your breakfast routine—whether you sit down at home or grab it on the go—and keep you satisfied until your next meal.

## Sweet-Potato Hash-Brown Frittata

This recipe is one for the weekend and can easily be sliced up and taken for breakfast on the go on a weekday. Packed with a variety of nutrients, it'll make you feel satisfied all morning.

**Yield:** 4 servings

**Time:** 1 hour

### Ingredients

1 extra-large (2 medium) sweet potato, shredded

9 large eggs, *divided*

Salt and cracked black pepper

1 onion, sliced

1 courgette (zucchini), sliced into half-moons

200 g (1 ¾ cups) mushrooms, sliced

100 g (3 cups) spinach, loosely packed

100 g (1 ¼ cups) feta (or cheddar)

### Method

1. Preheat the oven to 180ºC (350ºF).

2. Shred the sweet potato and press the liquid out using a cheesecloth or paper towel.

3. In a mixing bowl, combine the sweet potato with 1 whisked egg. Season with salt and pepper.

4. Transfer the mixture into a non-stick (or well-oiled) ovenproof skillet or dish. We recommend using a cast-iron skillet. Pat the mixture into the bottom and sides to create a crust, being careful to not leave any gaps.

5. Bake the sweet-potato mixture for 15 to 20 minutes or until slightly golden.

6. While the sweet potato is baking, prep your vegetables. In a mixing bowl, combine the remaining eggs, onion, courgette, mushrooms, and spinach.

7. When the sweet-potato crust is ready, pour the egg mixture into the skillet and bake for 30 minutes (or until the centre is firm).

8. Top the skillet with feta and return it to the oven for 5 to 10 minutes, until the cheese is melted and starting to crisp.

9. Let cool before slicing.

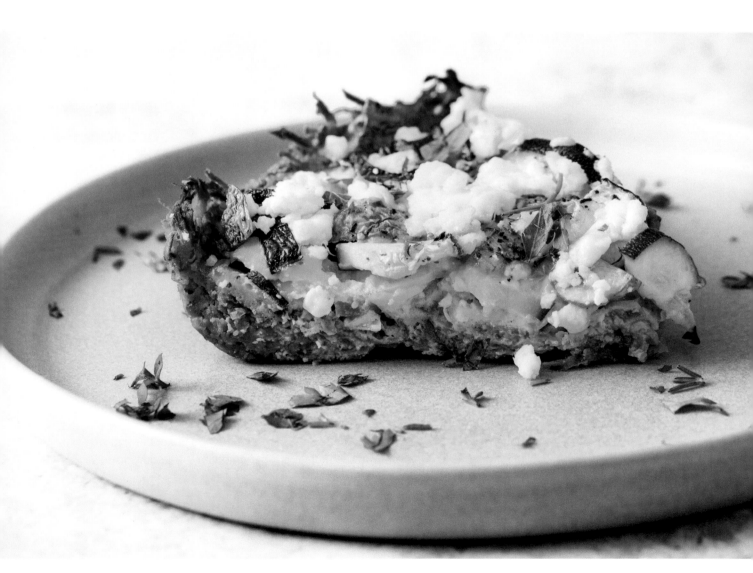

# Porridge With Chia-Seed Jam

Is there anything more comforting than a bowl of oats in the morning? We think not. Especially when you top it with our homemade chia-seed jam.

**Yield:** 1 serving (porridge); 2 servings (jam)

**Time:** 20 minutes

## Ingredients

**Chia-Seed Jam**

100 g (1 cup) frozen raspberries

3 tbsp maple syrup

2 ½ tbsp chia seeds

**Porridge**

50 g (½ cup) oats

150 mL (1 cup) milk

1 scoop protein powder, approx. 25 g (optional)

1 handful pumpkin seeds (optional)

## Method for the Jam

1. Begin by placing the frozen berries and maple syrup in a saucepan on medium heat.

2. Stir gently, and you'll see the berries start to break down and become syrupy.

3. Mix in the chia seeds and stir occasionally for approximately 10 to 15 minutes.

4. Once the jam mixture begins to thicken, remove it from the heat and leave it to cool for 5 minutes.

5. Serve the jam warm with the porridge. You can save half the jam by transferring the jam to a jar and leave it in the fridge. This will last up to two weeks in the fridge.

## Method for the Porridge

1. Heat the milk in a small saucepan over a high heat and add the oats. Stir for 4 to 5 minutes until you see little bubbles, then remove from heat. Stir in the protein powder and pour into a bowl to serve with the jam.

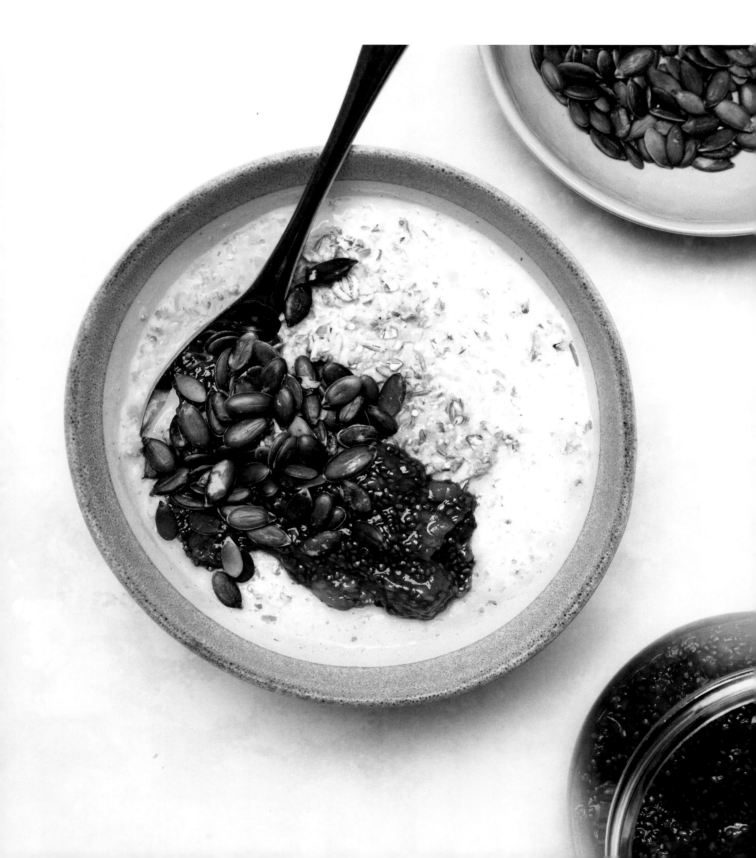

# Apple-Cinnamon Breakfast Bars

These are the ultimate grab-and-go breakfast bars. If you have a busy week ahead, make a batch on Sunday and keep them in the fridge to take out before work.

**Yield:** 6 bars

**Time:** 45-55 minutes

## Ingredients

100 g (1 cup) rolled oats

90 g (¾ cup) whole-wheat flour (plain or self-raising)

70 g (⅓ cup) plus 1 tbsp brown sugar, *divided*

4 tbsp melted ghee (or coconut oil)

4 tbsp water

1 tsp plus extra sprinkle of cinnamon, *divided*

1 tsp vanilla essence

1 medium apple, cut into thin slices

## Method

1. Preheat the oven to 180ºC (350ºF).

2. Prepare a 20x25 cm (8x10 inch) baking tray that's 5 to 8 cm (2 to 3 inches) deep (measurements approximate) by placing baking paper in the tray.

3. In a bowl, combine the oats, flour, and 70 g brown sugar.

4. Add the melted ghee, water, 1 tsp cinnamon, and vanilla essence and mix until all ingredients are combined together.

5. Set aside ½ cup of this mixture and use the rest to line the baking tray. You can use your hands to spread the crust evenly in the tray.

6. Cover the top of the crust with the thin apple slices. Then sprinkle with 1 tbsp brown sugar and finish off with a sprinkle of cinnamon.

7. Spread the reserved crust mix across the top.

8. Bake in the oven for 35 to 40 minutes.

9. Once the bars are baked, it's important to let them cool for about 15 minutes as they'll harden slightly whilst cooling.

10. Once they're cool, you can remove them from the tray, allow them to cool for 10 more minutes, and then cut evenly into squares.

11. Note: these bars should be stored in the fridge (in a container or wrapped in cling film) and will last approximately five days. You may also freeze these bars by wrapping them in cling film and storing in the freezer.

# Fluffy American Pancakes

Who doesn't love good old-fashioned pancake recipes! With all the 'healthy' alternative pancake recipes out there, we thought we'd take you back to the basics so you can whip up a batch on the weekend to share with the family (or have to yourself).

**Yield:** 2 to 4 servings

**Time:** 30 minutes

## Ingredients

190 g (1 ½ cups) plain flour

1 tsp baking powder

½ tsp salt

2 tbsp white granulated sugar

130 mL (½ cup) milk

1 large egg, lightly beaten

2 tbsp melted butter (allowed to cool, slightly)

Butter or oil for the skillet

Chocolate chips (optional)

Fresh or frozen berries (optional)

Maple syrup or golden syrup (optional)

## Method

1. Combine the flour, baking powder, salt, and sugar into a large mixing bowl.

2. In a separate bowl, mix together the milk, egg, and melted butter.

3. Pour the liquid mixture into the dry-ingredient mixture, stir to incorporate, and mix until smooth.

4. Let the batter sit for 10 to 15 minutes.

5. Heat a nonstick skillet over medium heat. Add butter or oil so the pancakes don't stick.

6. Add a ladle (or two, depending on the size of the pan) of batter. When the pancake starts to bubble and the sides become cooked, flip the pancakes to cook the other side.

7. Cook until both sides are golden brown.

8. Repeat steps 6 and 7 until all the batter is used up.

9. Top with any desired toppings. (We recommend chocolate chips with maple syrup.)

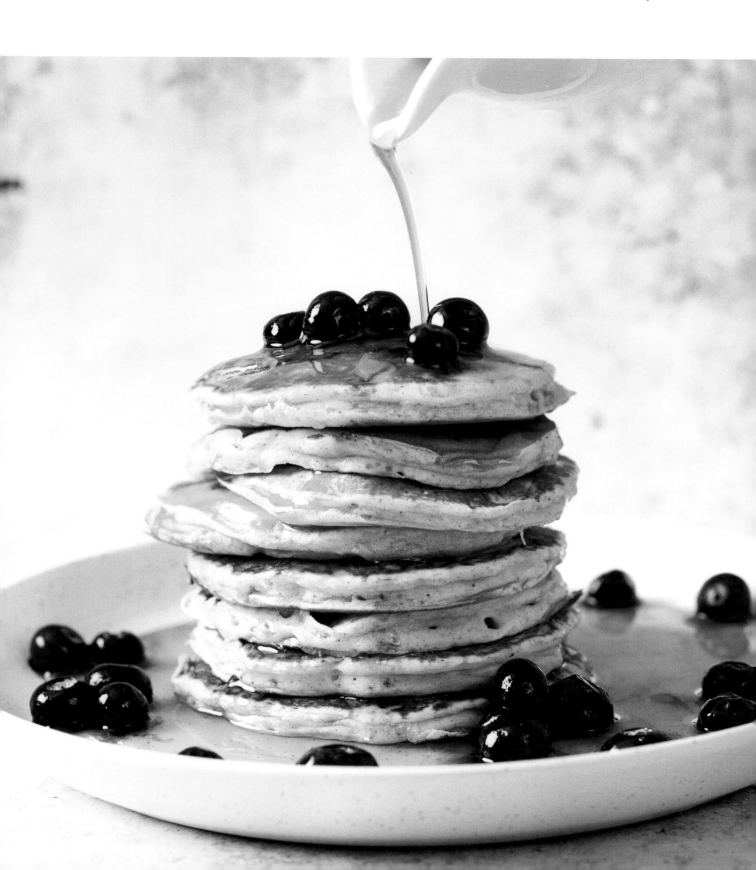

# Matcha Granola

Granola is a fun way to mix some nuts and seeds and add extra fibre to your breakfast bowl. We use matcha (Sophie's favourite), but you can use cacao powder instead, and it's just as tasty. We recommended serving this with some fruit and yoghurt or using it as a smoothie topper.

**Yield:** 6 servings

**Time:** 25 minutes

## Ingredients

300 g (2 cups) jumbo oats

100 g (1 cup) raw pistachios

140 g (1 cup) raw almonds

75 g (1 cup) coconut flakes

120 g (½ cup) pumpkin seeds

25 g (¼ cup) matcha green tea powder (can substitute cacao powder for matcha to make chocolate granola)

12 tbsp maple syrup (or honey) – ¾ cup (180 mL)

8 tbsp coconut oil, melted

## Method

1. Preheat the oven to 160℃ (320℉).

2. Line a baking tray with baking paper and set aside until the granola is mixed.

3. In a bowl, mix together the oats, pistachios, almonds, coconut flakes, pumpkin seeds, and matcha powder.

4. Pour the maple syrup and coconut oil into the bowl and mix well until all ingredients are combined.

5. Transfer the granola mix onto the prepared baking tray with baking paper.

6. Bake in the oven for 15 to 20 minutes, checking it halfway through to toss around on the baking sheet.

# Avocado Toast With Jammy Eggs

Did you know eggs have been labelled one of the most nutritious foods in the world? They contain a variety of different nutrients, and we think they taste best with avocado and toast. And in case you were wondering what a "jammy egg" is, it's a soft-boiled egg with a slightly congealed yolk, and it's delicious!

**Yield:** 1 serving

**Time:** 10 minutes

## Ingredients

2 eggs

2 slices sourdough bread

½ avocado, peeled, pitted, and sliced or mashed

Mixed seeds and seasonings (optional)

Chopped parsley (optional)

## Method

1. Bring a small or medium saucepan with water to a boil (Special tip: add a splash of white vinegar).

2. Once the water is boiling, add the eggs carefully and let them cook for 7 minutes.

3. While the eggs are cooking, toast the bread.

4. Arrange the sliced avocado on top of the toast.

5. Once the eggs are done, run them under cold water to stop the cooking process.

6. Peel the eggs and slice them down the middle.

7. Put the jammy eggs on top of the avocado toast and top with your preferred seasonings.

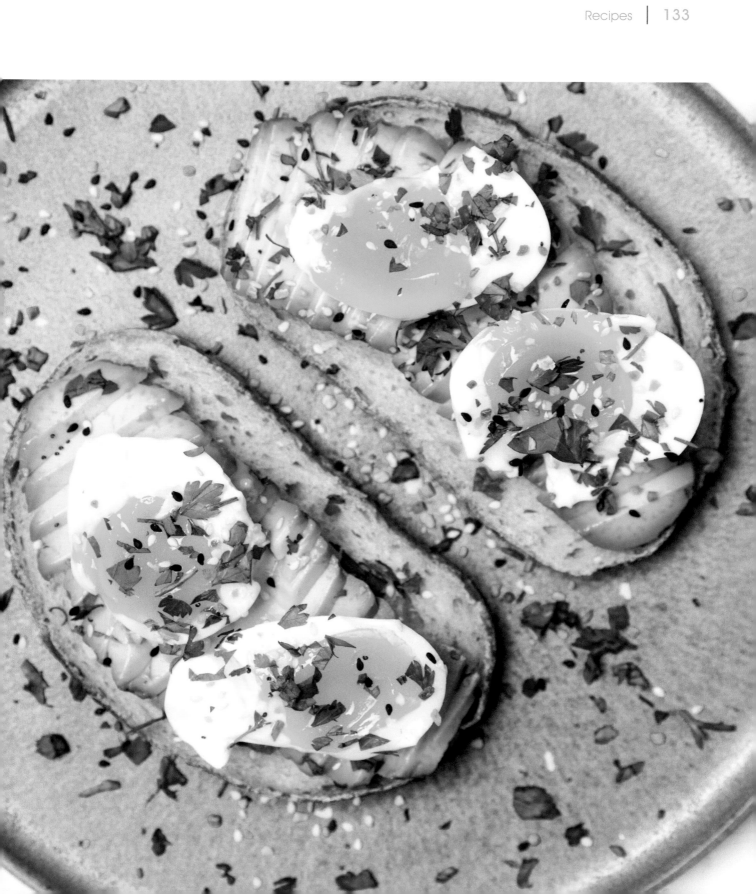

# Build-Your-Own Smoothie

Instead of giving you a specific smoothie recipe, we thought we'd break it down so you can build one based on your own preferences. Smoothies are a great option for those who don't always feel like eating first thing in the morning.

**Yield:** 1 serving

**Time:** 5 minutes

## Method

1. Choose a base: 250 mL (1 cup) soya, almond, oat, or coconut milk. (You can also use water if you don't want it milky.)

2. Make it creamy with one or more of these ingredients: banana, avocado, mango, coconut meat, and oats.

3. Add more fruits and veggies: berries, peach, pineapple, spinach, kale.

4. Add some protein: nut butter, chia seeds, protein powder.

5. Thicken it up with some ice (optional).

6. Blend and enjoy!

# Sweet-Potato Bowl

If you haven't turned your sweet potato into a sweet, sweet potato yet, you're missing out!

**Yield:** 1 serving

**Time:** 50 minutes

## Ingredients

1 medium sweet potato

1 tbsp nut butter

2 tbsp Greek yoghurt

Handful of fresh or frozen berries

sprinkle of seeds (optional)

drizzle of maple syrup (optional)

## Method

1. Preheat the oven to 180°C (350°F).

2. Use a knife to pierce a few holes in the sweet potato.

3. Cook in the oven for 45 minutes until very soft.

4. Once cooked, cut it in half and place both halves in a bowl.

5. Fill the sweet potato with the nut butter, Greek yoghurt, berries, and any additional desired toppings.

# Carrot-Cake Breakfast Muffins

An easy and nutritious recipe to whip up and take on a busy day—perfect for snacking too.

**Yield:** 6 muffins

**Time:** 25 minutes

## Ingredients

100 g (1 cup) oats

1 tsp baking powder

1 tsp cinnamon

4 tbsp of maple syrup

125 mL (½ cup) almond milk

3 tbsp nut or seed butter

1 tsp vanilla extract

1 medium banana, mashed

1 medium carrot, grated

30 g (¼ cup) chopped walnuts

## Method

1.  Preheat the oven to 180°C (350°F) and line a muffin tin with six muffin cups.

2.  Add the oats, baking powder, and cinnamon to a bowl.

3.  Stir in the maple syrup, milk, nut butter, vanilla extract, and mashed banana until well combined.

4.  Stir in the grated carrot and nuts.

5.  Spoon the mixture evenly across the 6 muffin cups.

6.  Bake for 20 minutes.

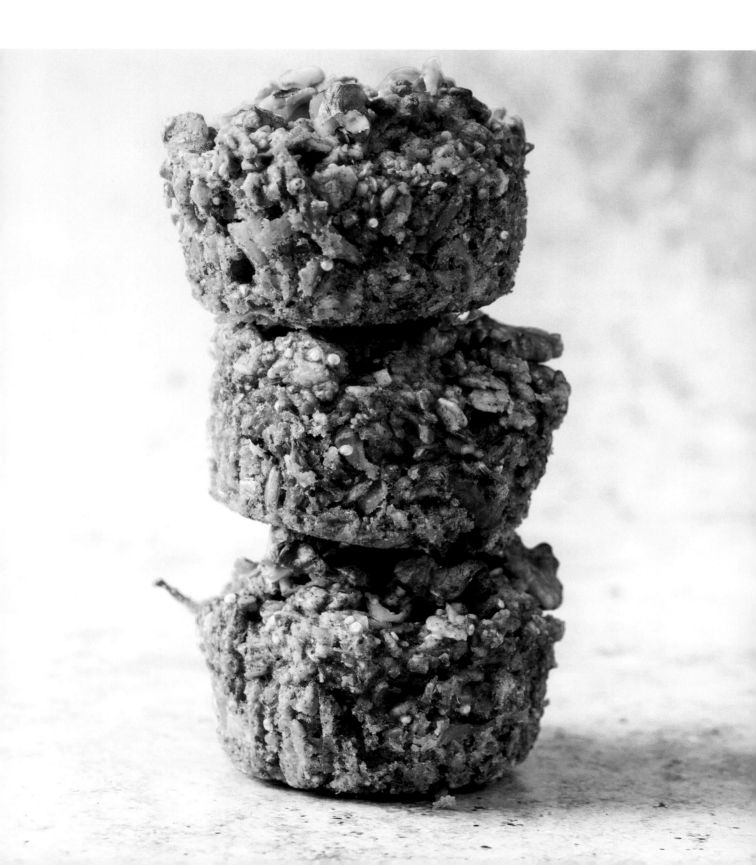

# Chai-Spiced Breakfast Quinoa

Switch up your usual porridge oat bowl for this aromatic quinoa bowl. Quinoa is also a complete protein, so it makes for a great vegan breakfast option.

**Yield:** 1 serving

## Ingredients

1 chai tea bag

130 mL (½ cup) almond milk

125 g (¾ cup) quinoa, cooked

½ tsp cinnamon

1 tbsp nut butter

Handful of blueberries

Sprinkle of pumpkin seeds

## Method

1. Heat the milk in a saucepan and soak the tea bag in the milk for a few minutes.

2. Add the quinoa and stir for a few minutes, then remove the tea bag from the pan.

3. Pour the tea into a bowl and top with the cinnamon, nut butter, blueberries, and pumpkin seeds.

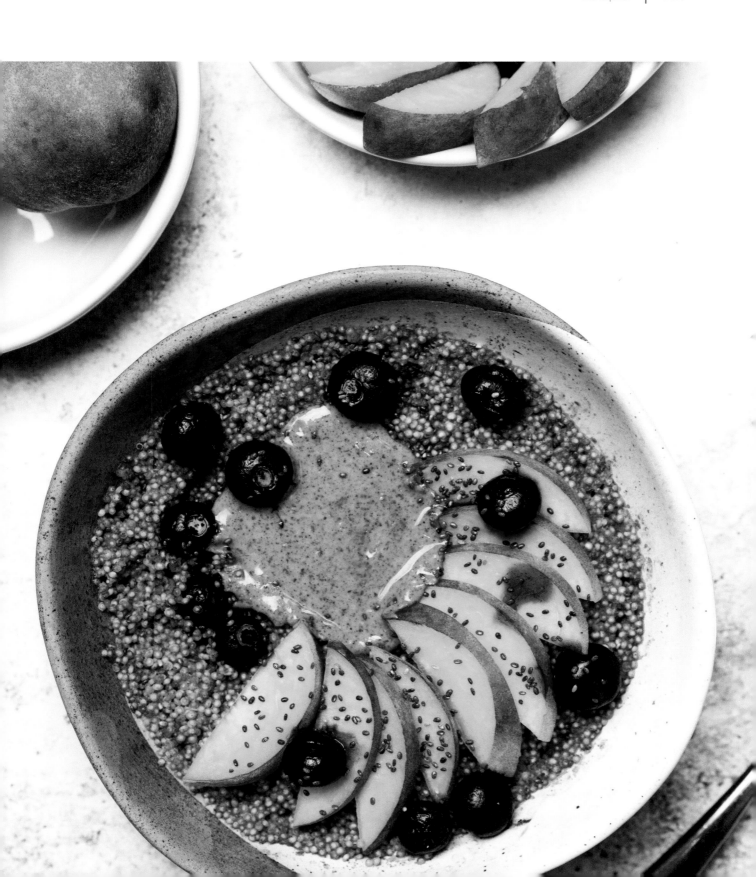

# Sweet-or-Savoury Omelette

Can you guess who prefers sweet and who likes the savoury option? Spoiler: Sophie is all about a sweet breakfast, and Bari usually prefers a savoury one. So take your pick.

**Yield:** 1 serving

**Time:** 5-10 minutes

## Ingredients

**Omelette**

2 or 3 eggs

Olive oil

**Savoury Toppings**

Handful of spinach

1 heaping tbsp of crumbled feta cheese

**Sweet Toppings**

60 g (½ cup) blueberries

1 tbsp nut butter

Method

1.  Whisk the eggs together.

2.  Heat the olive oil in a pan over medium-high heat.

3.  Pour the whisked eggs into the pan and allow to cook for 3 to 5 minutes.

4.  If having it savoury, add the spinach and feta on top approximately 1 minute before removing from the heat.

5.  Once cooked, slide the omelette onto a plate and add the blueberries and nut butter if you've opted for sweet.

# Lunch and Lunch Boxes

We've come up with some easy recipes that are perfect to pack into a lunch box because we're aware that some people find it challenging to build a satisfying packed lunch. We also have recipes that can be whipped up whilst working from home.

## Quinoa Greek Salad With Falafel

Dedicate some time on the weekend to whip this one up, and you'll have your lunch boxes for most of the week. It's delicious, well balanced, and packed with variety.

**Yield:** 4 servings

**Time:** 45 minutes

### Ingredients

**Falafel**

3 cloves garlic

2 (400 g or 15 oz.) tins chickpeas, rinsed and drained

135 g (1 ½ cups) rolled oats

2 heaping tbsp tahini

Juice of 1 large lemon

1 large egg plus 1 egg white

45 g (1 ½ cups) fresh parsley, packed, not chopped

75 g (1 ½ cups) fresh coriander (cilantro), packed, not chopped

1 ½ tbsp cumin

2 tsp turmeric

2 tsp chilli powder

½ tsp salt

1 tsp cracked black pepper

**Quinoa Greek Salad**

90 g (½ cup) quinoa, uncooked

1 cucumber, chopped

200 g (1 cup) cherry tomatoes, sliced

2 bell peppers, chopped

1 radish, sliced

100 g (½ cup) kalamata olives, sliced

100 g (1 cup) feta, crumbled

1 bunch fresh parsley, roughly chopped

1 bunch fresh mint, roughly chopped

1 tbsp dried oregano

1 ½ tbsp red wine vinegar

2 tbsp extra-virgin olive oil

## Method

1. Preheat the oven to 200°C (400°F).

2. Add all the falafel ingredients to a food processor. We recommend starting with the whole cloves of garlic to make sure they're chopped finely.

3. Once the batter is thick, scoop evenly sized falafel balls onto a baking-paper-lined baking tray. We recommend using a small ice-cream scoop to ensure a consistent size.

4. Bake for 30 minutes, flipping them halfway through.

5. While the falafel is baking, start on the quinoa salad. Cook quinoa according to packet instructions and let cool before adding it to the rest of the salad ingredients.

6. In a large mixing bowl, combine all the chopped salad ingredients, including the fresh and dried herbs, vinegar, and oil.

7. Once the quinoa has cooled, mix with the salad and top with the falafel.

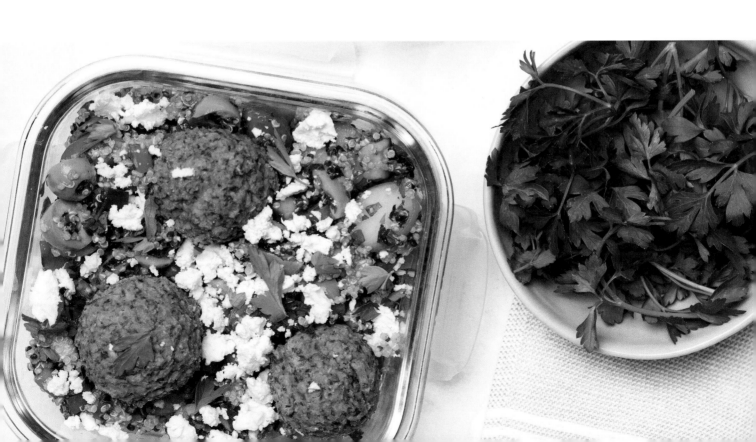

# Freekeh Caprese Salad

This is an incredibly refreshing and high-protein vegetarian salad that'll leave you feeling both full and satisfied. It's best enjoyed on the coast of Italy, but packed in a lunch box for the office is also encouraged!

**Yield:** 2 servings

**Time:** 45 minutes

## Ingredients

75 g (⅓ cup) raw freekeh

200 g (2 cups) fresh mozzarella, sliced

200 g (1 cup) cherry tomatoes, sliced

1 cucumber, deseeded and sliced

1 bunch fresh basil, roughly chopped

Salt and cracked black pepper

½ tbsp balsamic vinegar

1 tbsp extra-virgin olive oil

## Method

1. Cook the freekeh according to pack instructions.

2. Let the freekeh cool completely before mixing it with the other ingredients. To speed up the process, use precooked freekeh.

3. Combine the cooled freekeh, mozzarella, tomatoes, cucumber, and basil in a large mixing bowl.

4. Season with salt and pepper and drizzle with balsamic vinegar and extra-virgin olive oil before serving.

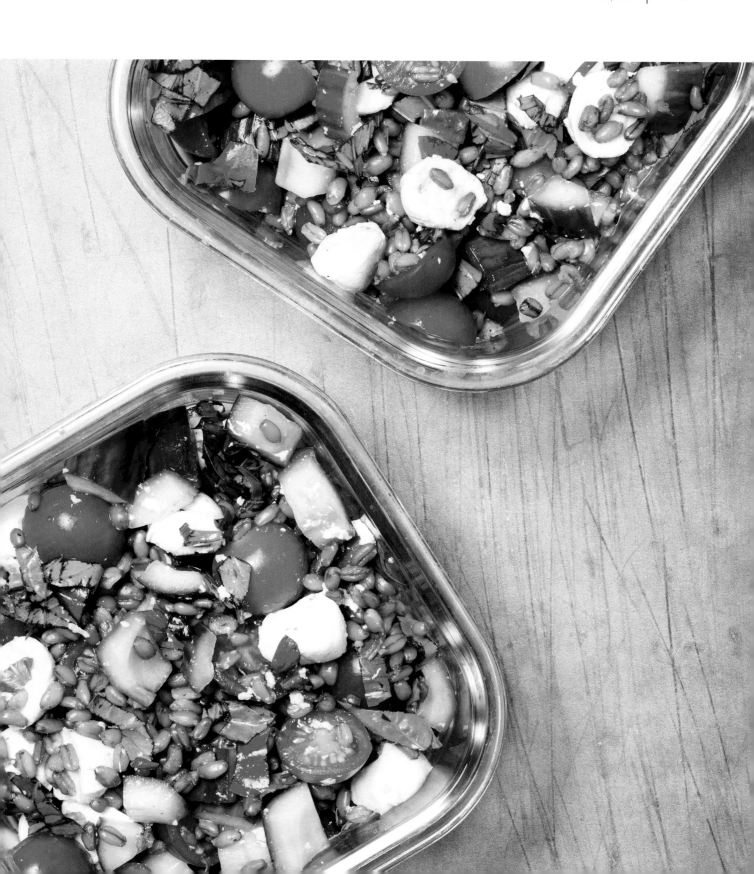

# Sweet-Potato and Black-Bean Burgers

This is the first recipe we ever made together, so we felt it absolutely necessary to include it in our book. Having now made these burgers many times, we rarely use a food processor because we like a chunky veggie burger. If you like your ingredients well blended, we recommended blending it—you decide!

**Yield:** 4 large or 8 small burgers

**Time:** 1 hour 45 minutes

## Ingredients

180 g (1 cup) quinoa, uncooked

1 (400 g or 15 oz.) tin black beans, rinsed and drained, *divided*

2 large sweet potatoes, cooked

2 eggs (regular or flaxseed eggs)

2 tbsp nutritional yeast (optional)

3 tbsp spicy-and-smoky spice blend (mix of cumin, onion powder, turmeric, chilli powder, salt, pepper, coriander, and cayenne pepper)

75 g (1 cup) chopped coriander (cilantro)

1 tbsp garlic powder

90 g (1 cup) rolled oats

Lettuce (optional)

Sauce of your choice (optional)

Bun (optional)

## Method

1. Preheat the oven to 180°C (350°F).

2. Make quinoa per packet instructions. For extra flavour, cook with either vegetable or chicken stock.

3. Place half the black beans in the food processor and reserve half for later.

4. Add the cooked sweet potatoes, eggs, nutritional yeast, herbs, and spices to the food processor and mix.

5. Move mixture to a large bowl and add reserved beans, oats, and quinoa, mixing until the batter is thick.

6. Place batter in the fridge for 1 hour for batter to set.

7. Place the burgers on parchment paper and bake in the oven for 20 to 30 minutes, flipping them halfway through. (Or you may cook the burgers on the hob if you wish.)

8. Add to your lunch box or enjoy with lettuce and sauce on a burger bun.

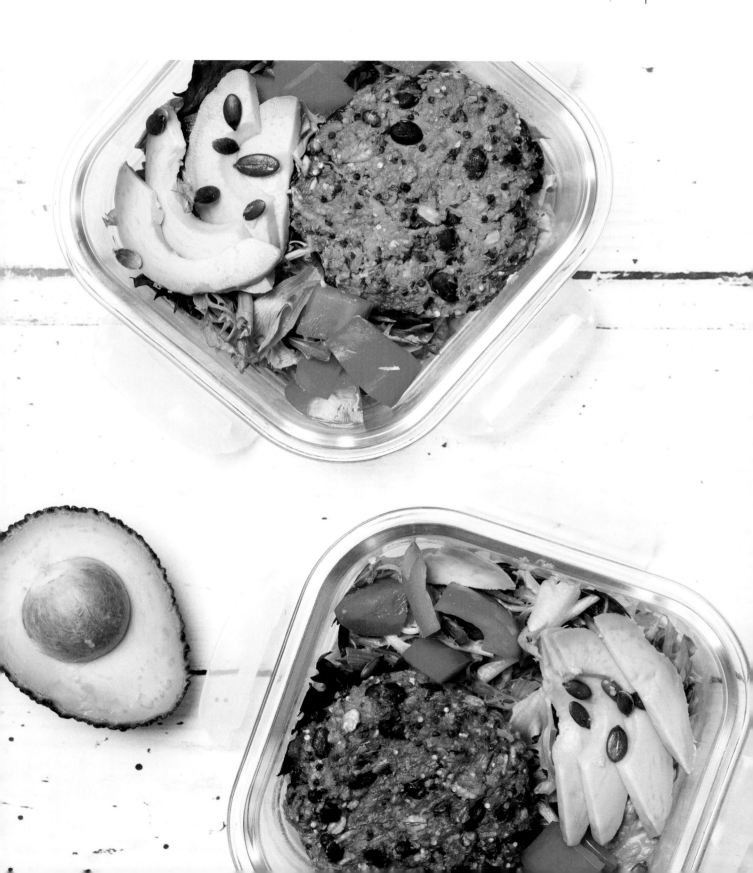

# Mixed-Bean Chilli

This is one for the whole family. This fibre-rich veggie chilli is made from mainly cupboard foods, so it's easy and cheap to make.

**Yield:** 4 servings

**Time:** 45 minutes

## Ingredients

Olive oil

1 medium onion (red or white), finely chopped

1 large carrot, finely chopped

1 red pepper, finely chopped

Salt to taste

1 (400 g or 15 oz.) tin chopped tomatoes

4 tbsp tomato paste or puree

3 tsp chilli powder

1 tsp cumin

Pepper to taste

½ tsp garlic powder

120 mL (½ cup) water

2 tbsp flaxseed (optional)

2 (400 g or 15 oz.) tins mixed beans or 1 (400 g) tin black beans and 1 (400 g) tin pinto beans

Coriander (cilantro), for garnish

Cooked brown rice

Cheddar cheese

Spring onions (scallions)

## Method

1. In a large pot, add oil and heat over medium heat.

2. Add the onion and cook for 6 minutes, stirring often. Add the carrot, red pepper, and a dash of salt.

3. Stir for 2 to 3 minutes, then add the tinned tomatoes, tomato paste, chili powder, cumin, garlic powder, and a dash of pepper.

4. Continue to cook for about 4 to 5 minutes, then pour in the beans, water, and flaxseed, if using.

5. Reduce to a low heat and simmer for 20 minutes.

6. Garnish with coriander and serve with cheddar cheese and spring onions over brown rice.

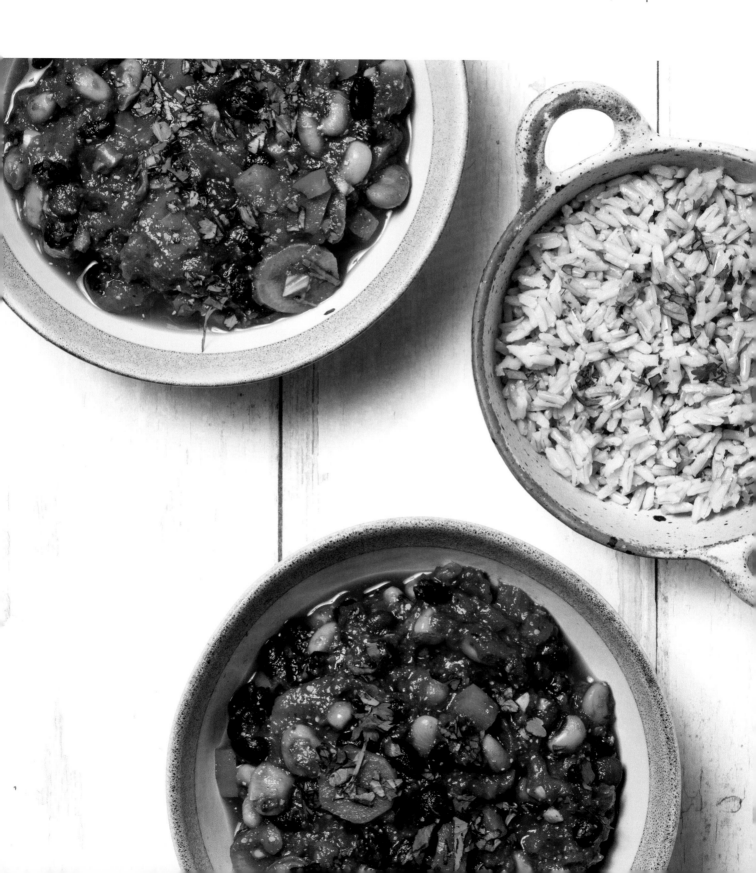

# Spicy Curry Lentil Soup

Soups are an easy way to add a little more nutrition in to your day and you add pretty much anything to them. #leftovers!

**Yield:** 4 servings

**Time:** 1 hour

## Ingredients

2 tbsp coconut oil

1 large onion, diced

3 cloves garlic, minced

1 (8 cm or 3 inch) piece fresh ginger, minced

1 ½ tbsp hot curry powder

½ tsp hot chilli powder (optional)

200 g (1 cup) split red lentils

1 x 400 mL (14 oz.) tin coconut milk

1 x 400 mL (14 oz.) tin crushed tomatoes

1 L vegetable stock

1 ½ tsp salt (more to taste)

Cracked black pepper to taste

200 g (1 cup) fresh spinach

Juice of 1 lime

1 tbsp Greek yoghurt (optional)

1 bunch fresh coriander, roughly chopped (optional)

## Method

1. Heat the coconut oil in a large stockpot or dutch oven over medium heat.

2. Add the onions and sauté until translucent.

3. Add the garlic and ginger and stir to prevent burning, for about 5 minutes.

4. Add the curry powder and chilli powder and stir to incorporate. Keep stirring to avoid burning the spices.

5. Add the lentils, coconut milk, tomatoes, stock, salt, and pepper

6. Bring the mixture to a boil and then simmer for 30 to 40 minutes, stirring occasionally.

7. Add the spinach and lime juice.

8. Top with Greek yoghurt and fresh coriander if desired.

# Ten-Minute Pizza Bagels

This is one of our favourite quick and satisfying at-home lunch recipes. Minimal ingredients are needed, and it's well balanced and deliciously cheesy. We like seeded wholemeal bagels for extra fibre.

**Yield:** 2 servings

**Time:** 10 minutes

## Ingredients

2 bagels

4 tbsp tomato puree

70 g (¾ cup) grated cheese

Handful of spinach

## Method

1. Cut your bagels in half and toast them in a toaster very lightly.

2. Once toasted, spread 1 tbsp tomato puree per half bagel.

3. Top with grated cheese and spinach leaves.

4. Place on foil on a baking tray and toast under the grill on medium heat until the cheese is melted and slightly crispy.

# Green Pesto Pasta

Sometimes we want chocolate—sometimes we want greens!

**Yield:** 2 servings

**Time:** 20 minutes

## Ingredients

170 g (¾ cup) fusilli pasta, uncooked

1 tbsp olive oil

2 cloves of garlic, minced

80 g (1 ½ cups) garden peas

160 g (1 ¼ cups) asparagus, chopped

2 tbsp green pesto (see our homemade recipe)

Salt and cracked black pepper to taste

## Method

1. Boil the pasta, following the instructions according to the pack.

2. Once cooked, remove from heat and drain, then rinse with cold water and set aside.

3. Heat the olive oil in a pan over medium heat and add the garlic, cooking for 2 minutes, until it turns golden.

4. Add the peas and asparagus to the pan and cook for a few more minutes. Add the fusilli and pesto and season with the salt and pepper.

5. Cook for a few more minutes, then serve.

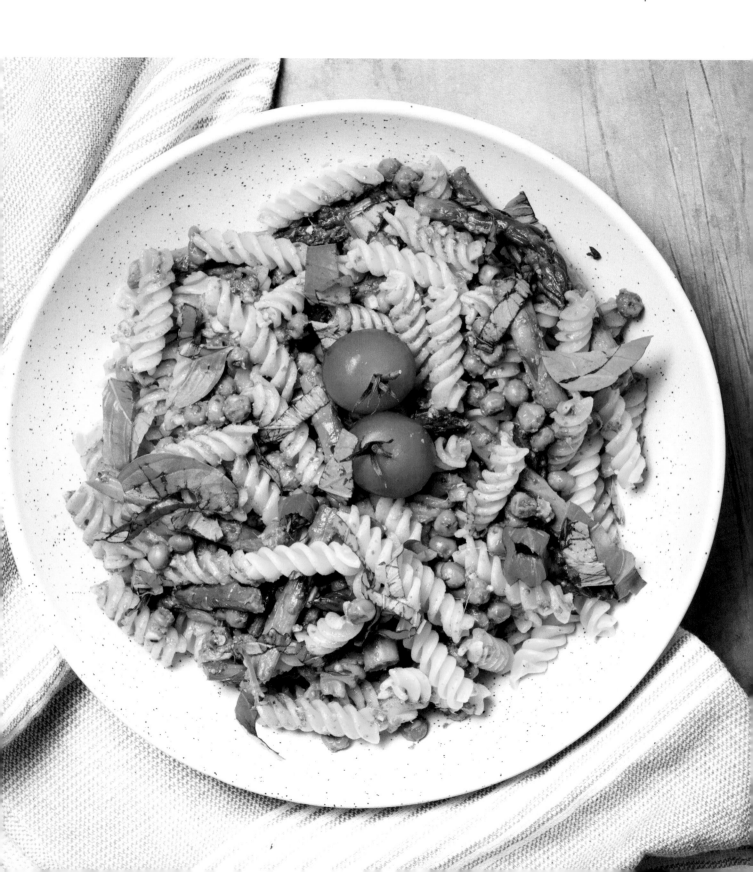

# Cheesy Courgette Fritters

We think courgette is best served with cheese. Fritters are a great way to use up leftovers or add extra veg to your diet.

**Yield:** 4 servings (2 fritters each)

**Time:** 15 minutes

## Ingredients

250 g (2 cups) grated courgette (zucchini), approximately 2 large courgettes

60 g (1 cup) panko bread crumbs

2 eggs

35 g (⅓ cup) grated cheddar cheese

28 g (¼ cup) finely shredded mozzarella cheese

Salt and cracked black pepper to taste

Olive oil

## Method

1. Place the grated courgette in a mesh bag (or you can also use your hands) and squeeze out as much of the liquid as you can.

2. Transfer the courgette to a bowl and add all other ingredients except olive oil.

3. Mix until well combined and heat the olive oil in a pan over medium heat.

4. Scoop out the mix evenly, using your hands to mould the fritters, and cook two to three fritters at a time (depending on size of pan).

5. Cook for about 5 minutes on each side, flipping them once.

6. You may need to add a little olive oil to the pan between batches.

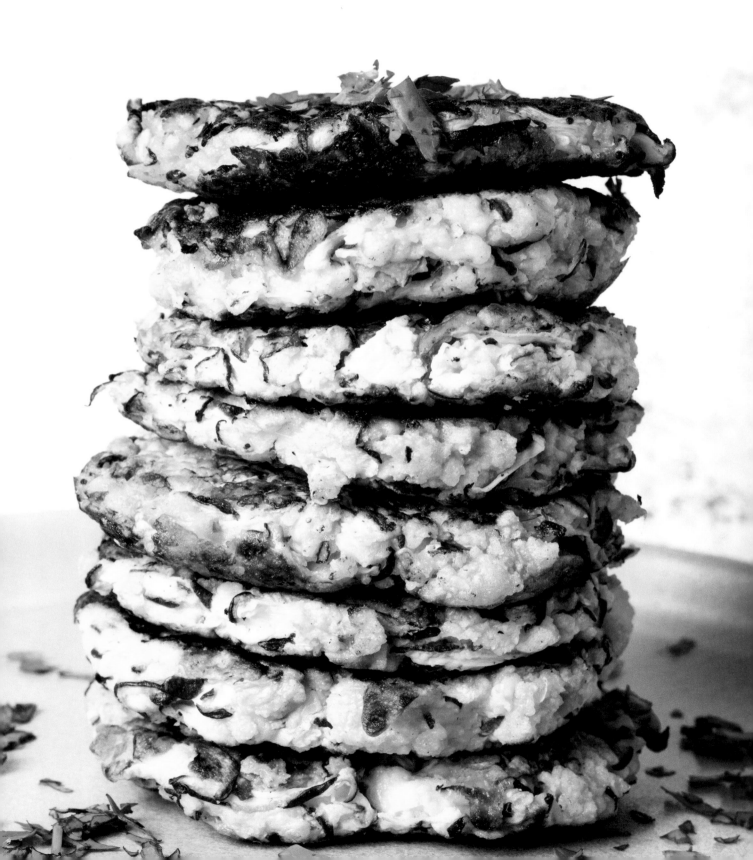

# Lentil and Butternut-Squash Salad

If you're looking for a budget-friendly and easy-to-make recipe—look no further!

**Yield:** 4 servings

**Time:** 30 minutes

## Ingredients

400 g (3 cups) butternut squash, cubed

1 tbsp olive oil

Salt and cracked black pepper to taste

120 g (1 ½ cups) rocket (arugula)

2 (400 g or 15 oz.) tins cooked lentils, rinsed and drained

120 g (½ cup) goat cheese, crumbled

## Method

1. Preheat the oven to 200°C (400°F).

2. Place the cubed butternut squash on a baking-paper-lined baking tray and toss with 1 tbsp olive oil.

3. Season with salt and pepper and bake for 20 minutes, flipping them halfway through.

4. While the butternut squash is cooking, toss the rocket with the lentils and add the goat cheese.

5. Add the warm butternut squash, adjust for seasoning, and serve.

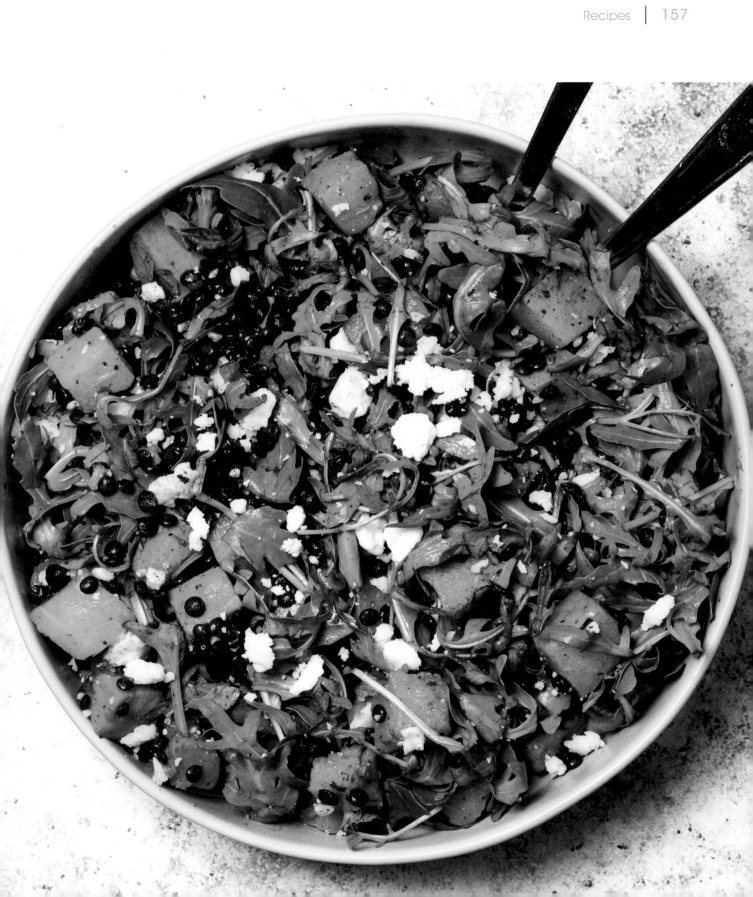

# Thai Tofu Salad With Edamame

Get your plant-based food diversity in with this recipe! Packed with a wide variety of plants, and a ton of flavour, this will leave your taste buds and gut microbiome very happy!

**Yield:** 4 servings

**Time:** 45 minutes

## Ingredients

400 g extra-firm tofu (1 large block)

1 tbsp corn flour

1 ½ tbsp olive oil

½ red cabbage, grated

2 large carrots, grated

1 cucumber, deseeded and sliced

2 bell peppers, sliced thin

200 g (1 cup) cherry tomatoes, halved

1 bunch fresh coriander (cilantro), roughly chopped

1 bunch fresh mint, roughly chopped

1 large spring onion (scallion), sliced thin

300 g (1 ½ cups) edamame beans, deshelled

1 tbsp sesame seeds

Peanut dressing (see recipe index)

1 large lime, sliced

## Method

1. Preheat the oven to 200°C (400°F).
2. Press excess liquid out of the tofu and slice into 3 cm (1 inch) cubes.
3. Place tofu on a baking-paper-lined baking sheet and cover with corn flour and olive oil.
4. Bake for 30 minutes, flipping them halfway through.
5. While the tofu is baking, prepare the salad in a large mixing bowl, adding the vegetables, tomatoes, and herbs.
6. Add the edamame beans, sesame seeds, and baked tofu.
7. Dress with the peanut dressing and serve with fresh lime.

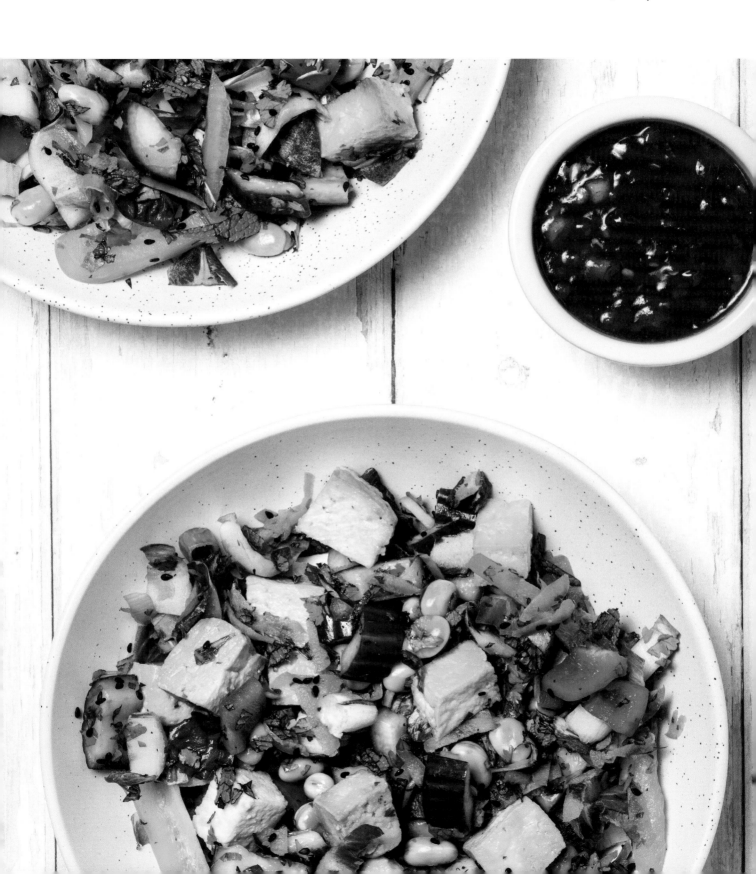

# Dinner

We're sharing a range of dinner recipes that have diverse ingredients and require no professional chef skills to make. Whether you're in need of quick, easy recipes or ones that require a little more time and care, we've got you covered. Being that we, Sophie and Bari, don't eat meat, we've included fish but no meat in the recipes; however, don't be afraid to switch out tofu for chicken if that's your thing.

## Bari's Chickpea, Sweet Potato, and Spinach Curry

This is one of Bari's favourite meals to batch cook or cook for friends. It also works great in a slow cooker.

**Yield:** 4 servings

**Time:** 1 hour

### Ingredients

2 medium sweet potatoes, cubed

1 ½ tbsp olive oil

Salt and cracked black pepper to taste

1 ½ tbsp coconut oil

1 medium onion, diced

3 cloves garlic, minced

5 cm (2 inch) cube ginger, minced

2 ½ tbsp garam masala

1 tsp cumin

1 tsp turmeric

2 tsp chilli powder 2 tbsp tomato paste

1 (400 g or 15 oz.) tin chopped tomatoes

1 x 400 mL (15 oz.) tin coconut milk

2 (400 g or 15 oz.) tins chickpeas, rinsed and drained

400 g (2 cups) spinach

1 large bunch coriander (cilantro), roughly chopped

Juice of 1 large lime

Additional coriander (optional), roughly chopped

## Method

1. Preheat the oven to 200°C (400°F).

2. Place the cubed sweet potato on a baking-paper-lined baking sheet and season with olive oil, salt, and pepper.

3. Bake for 30 minutes, flipping them halfway through.

4. In a large stockpot or dutch oven, heat the coconut oil over medium heat.

5. Add the onions and sauté until translucent.

6. Add the garlic and ginger and sauté until fragrant. Stir often to prevent burning.

7. Add the garam masala, cumin, turmeric, and chilli powder and stir to incorporate.

8. Season with salt and pepper.

9. Add the tomato paste, tinned tomatoes, and coconut milk.

10. Bring to a boil and then simmer for 30 minutes.

11. Add the chickpeas, spinach, cooked sweet potato, coriander, and lime juice.

12. Adjust seasonings to taste, top with additional coriander if desired, and serve.

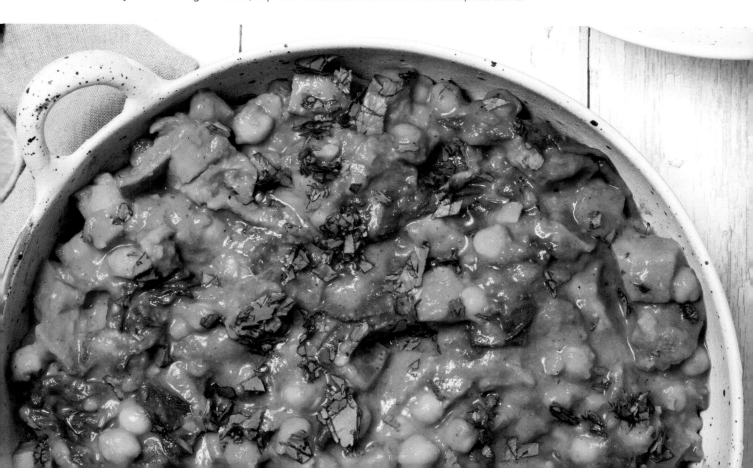

# Sophie's Pasta Bake

This is Sophie's signature dish—and also a sneaky way to add more veggies and plant foods to a meal.

**Yield:** 3 to 4 servings

**Time:** 30 minutes

## Ingredients

200 g (2 cups) dried red-lentil pasta

120 g (1 ¼ cups) mozzarella cheese (or grated mozzarella)

200 g (1 ¼ cups) broccoli

200 g (1 ¼ cups) green peas

400 g (1 ¾ cups) tomato-and-basil pasta sauce

1 (400 g or 15 oz.) tin black beans, rinsed and drained

1 (400 g or 15 oz.) tin chickpeas, rinsed and drained

## Method

1. Preheat the oven to 180°C (350°F). You'll need a large, oven-safe dish to hold the pasta.

2. Boil the pasta for 6 to 7 minutes (according to pack instructions) and stir often to prevent it from burning or sticking at the bottom. If using regular pasta, cooking time may be longer.

3. Whilst the pasta is boiling, cut the mozzarella into small slices and set aside.

4. Cut the broccoli into small florets and boil with the peas for 2 to 3 minutes.

5. Drain the pasta and rinse under cold water.

6. Pour the pasta into your oven-safe dish and stir in the pasta sauce.

7. Add the black beans and chickpeas to the pasta dish.

8. Add in the boiled broccoli and peas and then the prepared mozzarella.

9. Bake for 15 to 20 minutes, depending on how crispy you want the top of the pasta. (I like mine crispy.)

10. Remove the dish from the oven and serve up instantly. You can also save it and take it to work the next day—allow it to cool and keep it in an airtight container in the fridge until ready to eat.

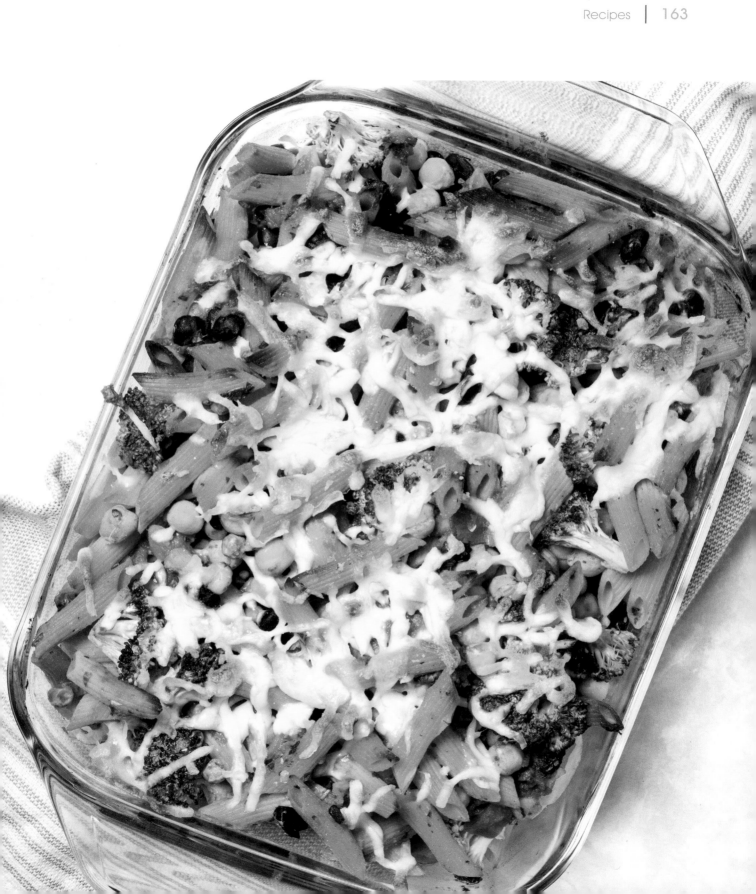

# Teriyaki Tofu Bowl

Buddha-bowl meals are a great way to add diversity to your diet. We've chosen simple ingredients here, but feel free to add any type of veggies and grains.

**Yield:** 2 servings

**Time:** 45 minutes

## Ingredients

200 g (1 block) extra-firm tofu

¼ cup corn flour

160 g (2 ¼ cups) broccoli

6 tbsp teriyaki sauce, *divided*

200 g (1 cup) cooked freekeh (or brown rice)

2 medium carrots, chopped

1 avocado, peeled, pitted, and sliced or chopped

4 tbsp sesame seeds

Method

1. Preheat the oven to 180°C (350°F) and line a baking tray with baking paper.

2. Cut the tofu into cubes, place in a bowl, and mix with the corn flour, tossing the cubes around so they're coated.

3. Place the tofu on the baking sheet.

4. Cut the broccoli into florets (don't cut too small) and place them next to the tofu on the baking sheet.

5. Cook for 25 minutes in the oven and then remove the broccoli and place in a bowl.

6. Toss the tofu and allow it to cook for 10–15 more minutes.

7. Add the tofu to a separate bowl.

8. Use half the teriyaki sauce, reserving the other half, and coat the tofu, tossing it round the bowl gently.

9. Divide into two portions and serve up, dividing the freekeh, broccoli, raw carrots, and avocado.

10. Use up the reserved teriyaki sauce (to be divided across each portion).

11. Sprinkle with sesame seeds.

# Lentil Spag Bowl

There are few things as cosy as a big bowl of pasta. This is a delicious and meat-free take on a traditional bolognese. Personally, as we add the red wine to the dish, we also pour ourselves a glass—cheers!

**Yield:** 4 servings

**Time:** 1 hour

## Ingredients

1 ½ tbsp olive oil

1 onion, finely chopped

1 large carrot, finely chopped

1 bell pepper, diced

100 g (1 ⅓ cups) mushrooms, finely chopped

1 courgette (zucchini), finely chopped

4 cloves garlic, minced

1 tbsp dried thyme

2 tbsp tomato paste

60 mL (¼ cup) red wine

1 tbsp worcestershire sauce

1 (400 g or 15 oz.) tin cooked lentils

2 (400 g or 15 oz.) tins crushed tomatoes

Salt and cracked black pepper to taste

200 g uncooked spaghetti

100 g (1 cup) parmesan cheese, grated

1 bunch fresh basil, roughly chopped

1 tbsp red chilli flakes (optional)

Extra parmesan cheese, grated (optional)

## Method

1. In a large skillet over medium heat, sauté the onions, carrots, and peppers in olive oil for 5 minutes.

2. Add the mushrooms and courgette and cook for another 5 to 7 minutes.

3. Add the garlic and dried thyme and sauté for 2 to 3 minutes.

4. Add the tomato paste, red wine, and worcestershire sauce and stir to incorporate well.

5. Add the lentils and mix well for 5 to 7 minutes.

6. Add the crushed tomatoes and season with salt and pepper.

7. Bring to a boil and then reduce the heat and let simmer for 25 to 30 minutes.

8.  Cook spaghetti according to the pack instructions.

9.  Add the 100 g parmesan cheese, fresh basil, and chilli flakes to the lentil mixture and adjust the seasoning.

10. Divide the cooked spaghetti amongst 4 portions and spoon the lentil mixture on top of each. Top with parmesan cheese if desired.

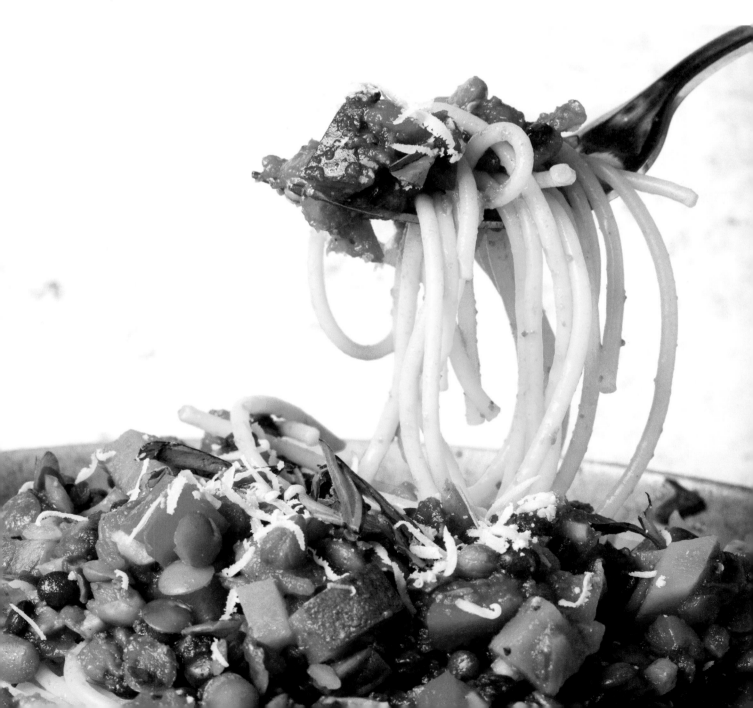

# Pesto Veggie, Chickpea, and Halloumi Tray Bake

We couldn't have a recipe book without a halloumi dish!

**Yield:** 2 to 3 servings

**Time:** 30 minutes

## Ingredients

400 g (2 cups) cherry tomatoes

1 red onion, sliced thick

1 (400 g or 15 oz.) tin chickpeas, rinsed, drained, and dried

2 tbsp olive oil

Salt and cracked black pepper

3 large handfuls kale, de-stemmed and chopped

225 g (1 block) halloumi, sliced thick

150 g (2/3 cups) classic pesto (see recipe index)

1 bell pepper, cut into thick chunks

1 courgette, cut into rounds

½ bunch fresh basil leaves, roughly chopped

Fresh sourdough (optional)

Additional pesto (optional)

## Method

1.  Preheat the oven to 200°C (400°F).

2.  Add the tomatoes, peppers, courgette, red onion, and chickpeas to a large baking dish.

3.  Season with olive oil, salt, and cracked black pepper and roast for 15 minutes.

4.  Remove the tray, add the kale, and mix. Cook for 5 extra minutes.

5.  While the veggies are baking, grill the halloumi on medium heat in a nonstick skillet until both sides are golden.

6.  Remove and top with halloumi, pesto, and fresh basil.

7.  Serve with a fresh sourdough and extra pesto for a delicious meal.

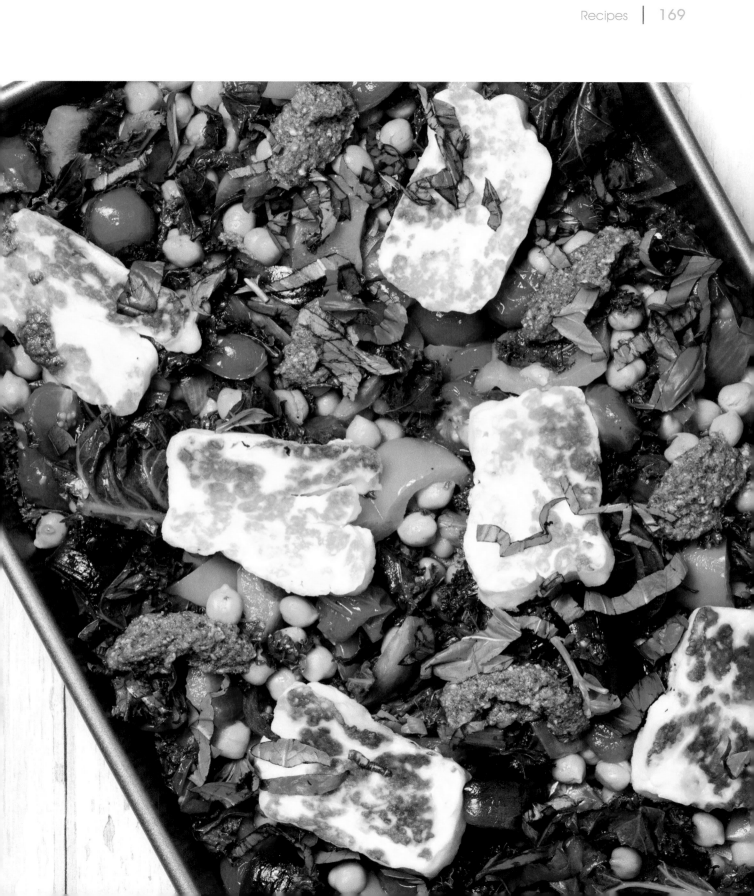

# Miso Salmon

Miso is one of our favourite flavours to use in cooking. We feel it works perfectly with salmon, but you can use any fish.

**Yield:** 1 serving

**Time:** 25 minutes

## Ingredients

1 tbsp white miso

1 tbsp soya sauce

1 tbsp maple syrup

1 tbsp water

½ tsp ground ginger

1 salmon fillet

Avocado oil

80 g (½ cup) asparagus

125 g (½ cup) brown rice (cooked weight)

## Method

1. Preheat the oven to 180°C (350°F).

2. In a small bowl, create the miso glaze by mixing together the miso, soya sauce, maple syrup, water, and ginger.

3. Place the salmon fillet (skin down) on foil or baking paper on a baking tray and marinade it with ½ the miso mix.

4. Cook for approximately 15 minutes.

5. Heat the avocado oil in a pan over medium heat and cook the asparagus, turning regularly for 5 to 6 minutes.

6. Serve the rice in a bowl and add the asparagus and salmon on top.

7. Use the rest of the miso glaze to marinade the salmon again once it's cooked.

8. Note: for a quick dish, pan fry the salmon with the greens and marinade (see photo).

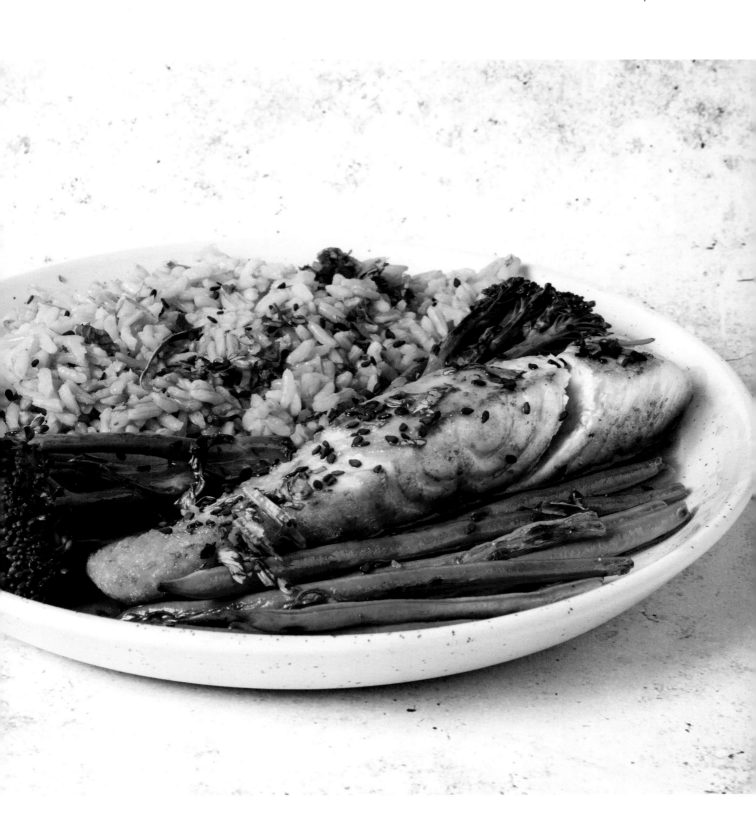

# Quinoa-Crusted Tofu Nuggets

Pimp up your tofu with our quinoa-crusted nuggets—just four ingredients and easy to make.

**Yield:** 2 servings

**Time:** 30 minutes

## Ingredients

200 g (1 block) extra-firm tofu

90 g (½ cup) cooked quinoa

1 tbsp chia seeds

Bottle of sticky BBQ sauce

Leafy greens and veggies

## Method

1. Preheat the oven to 180°C (350°F) and line a baking tray with baking paper.

2. Make sure the tofu is drained of any water, and cut into thick slices, making nugget shapes.

3. Mix the quinoa and chia seeds in a bowl.

4. Generously dip each tofu nugget into BBQ sauce, then coat with the quinoa mix and place on the prepared baking tray.

5. Cook for 15 to 20 minutes, until nice and crispy.

6. Serve up with some leafy greens and veg add to your lunch box.

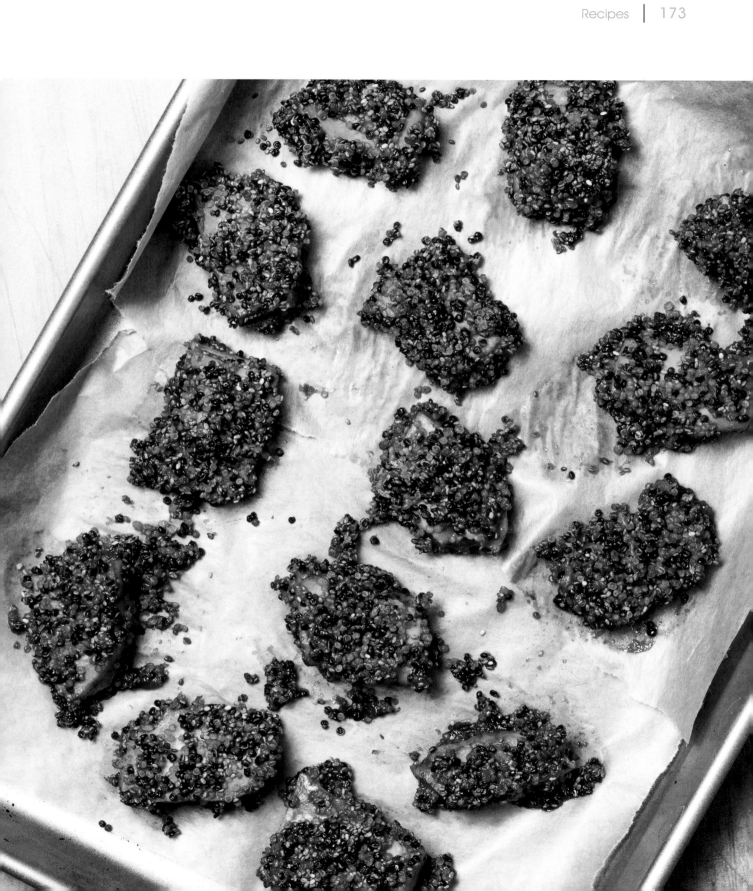

# Tomato Cod Bake

This bake is a very classic yet very flavourful dish to cook for the whole family.

**Yield:** 4 servings

**Time:** 45 minutes

## Ingredients

**Tomato Mixture**

1 tbsp olive oil

1 medium onion, diced

2 cloves garlic, minced

200 g (1 cup) cherry tomatoes

60 mL (¼ cup) vegetable stock

60 mL (¼ cup) white wine

1 tbsp dried oregano

2 tbsp capers

2 tbsp fresh basil, roughly chopped

2 tbsp fresh parsley, roughly chopped

4 tbsp unsalted butter

Salt and cracked black pepper to taste

**Cod**

4 fillets fresh cod

Juice of 1 lemon

Salt and cracked black pepper

Olive oil

**Extras**

Cooked couscous (optional)

Steamed broccoli (optional)

Method

1. Preheat the oven to 200°C (400°F).

2. In a medium skillet, heat the olive oil over medium heat. Add the onion and garlic and sauté until garlic is fragrant and onions are translucent.

3. Add the tomatoes, vegetable stock, white wine, oregano, and capers and cook until the tomatoes start to break down and the mixture begins to thicken.

4. Remove from the heat and add the fresh herbs, butter, salt, and pepper.

5. Lightly oil a casserole dish and place the cod fillets in a single layer. Season with lemon juice, salt, and pepper.

6. Lightly drizzle with olive oil and then cover with aluminium foil.

7. Bake for 15 to 20 minutes.

8. Remove the foil and cover with the tomato mixture.

9. We recommend serving with a side of couscous and steamed broccoli.

# Prawn Stir-Fry With Noodles

Stir-fries are (in our opinion) one of the easiest meals to whip up, and you can throw in any leftovers you have sitting in the fridge too. You can add or omit ingredients based on what you like.

**Yield:** 2 servings

**Time:** 20 minutes

## Ingredients

100 g (1 cup) egg noodles, uncooked

1 tbsp olive oil

5 cm (2 inch) piece ginger, minced

2 cloves garlic, minced

1 onion, sliced

1 bell pepper, sliced

100 g (1 cup) mange-touts (snow peas)

1 tbsp soya sauce

1 tbsp oyster sauce

100 mL (½ cup) plus 1 tbsp vegetable stock

1 carrot, shredded

200 g (¾ cup) raw king prawn (shrimp)

100 g bean sprouts

100 g (1 cup) spinach

1 to 2 tsp corn flour if needed

2 spring onions (scallions), sliced

1 red chilli, sliced thin

1 tsp cold-pressed sesame oil

## Method

1. Cook the egg noodles according to pack instructions. Once cooked, slightly oil the noodles to prevent them from sticking.

2. Heat the olive oil in a wok or large frying pan over medium-high heat.

3. Add the ginger and garlic and sauté until fragrant.

4. Add the onion and pepper and stir to prevent from burning.

5. Add the mange-touts, soya sauce, oyster sauce, and vegetable stock and stir for a few minutes, then add the shredded carrots.

6. Add the prawn, bean sprouts, and spinach. Cook until the prawn is pink and opaque.

7. If the sauce in the stir-fry is runny, you can add 1 to 2 tsp corn flour.

8. Add the noodles to the vegetable-and-prawn mixture and incorporate.

9. Serve the stir-fry over the noodles and top with spring onions, sliced chillies, and a drizzle of sesame oil.

# Desserts

## Sophie's Salted-Caramel Brownies

An absolute must-make—we've yet to meet anyone who doesn't love these brownies. Think soft, gooey, and chocolaty.

**Yield:** 9 brownies

**Time:** 30 minutes

### Ingredients

200 g (7.1 oz.) of galaxy salted-caramel chocolate (or any block of salted-caramel chocolate), divided

170 g (¾ cup) melted butter

250 g (1 ¼ cups) castor sugar

2 eggs

2 tsp vanilla extract

95 g (¾ cup) plain flour

30 g (¼ cup) cacao or cocoa powder

### Method

1. Preheat the oven to 180°C (350°F). Line a 20x20 cm (8x8 inch) square baking tray with baking paper.

2. Break the chocolate bars into chunks.

3. Melt half of the chocolate in the microwave in 20-second intervals, saving the other half for later.

4. In a large bowl, mix the butter and sugar with an electric hand mixer, then beat in the eggs and vanilla for 1 to 2 minutes, until the mixture becomes fluffy and light in colour.

5. Whisk in the melted chocolate (make sure it's not too hot or else the eggs will cook)

6. Then sift in the flour and cocoa powder.

7. Fold in the flour and cocoa powder, being careful not to overmix as doing so will cause the brownies to be more cakelike in texture.

8. Fold in the reserved chocolate chunks, then transfer the batter to the prepared baking dish.

9. Bake for 20 to 25 minutes, depending on how fudgy you like your brownies. We baked our brownies shown in the photo for 22 minutes.

10. Enjoy warm or cool.

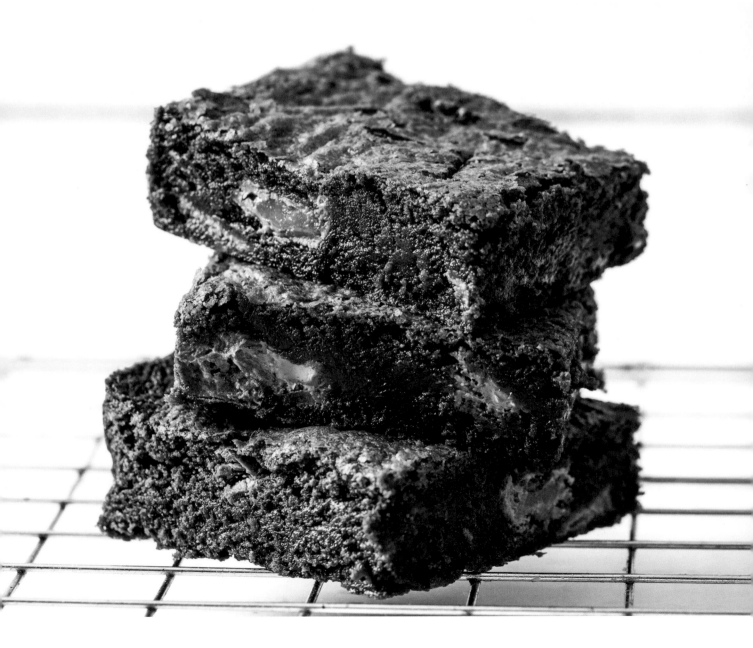

# Chocolate Avocado Mousse

This is a different take on a chocolate mousse. The avocado adds some essential fats and a creamier texture—and you wouldn't even know it's there.

**Yield:** 2 servings

**Time:** 1 hour 5 minutes

## Ingredients

1 large avocado, peeled, pitted, and chopped

4 tbsp maple syrup

50 g (½ cup) cacao or cocoa powder

60 mL (¼ cup) plus 1 tbsp almond milk

1 tsp vanilla paste or extract

## Method

1. Add all ingredients into a food processor and blend until smooth (scraping down the sides in between).

2. Transfer into serving dishes and cover with cling film.

3. Allow to chill in the fridge for 1 hour.

# Mug Cakes

Ever feel like having something sweet after your dinner but don't know what to have? Our mug cakes are easy to make and will satisfy your sweet tooth! Substitute the egg with a flaxseed egg for a vegan mug cake.

Each mug-cake recipe yields 1 serving.

## Ingredients

**Three-Ingredient Chocolate Mug Cake**

1 medium ripe banana, mashed

1 egg

2 tbsp cacao powder

**Six-Ingredient Peanut-Butter Mug Cake**

1 egg

2 tbsp peanut butter

2 tbsp plant-based milk

2 tbsp maple syrup

3 tbsp ground almonds (or ground oats)

1 tbsp chocolate chips

## Method

1. Blend in a blender all ingredients for your chosen mug cake.

2. Grease a mug with coconut oil and pour the mix into the mug.

3. Microwave for approximately 1 minute.

4. Enjoy!

# Bari's Lemon Shortbread Bars

A refreshing yet indulgent dessert! We recommend this one for a dinner party evening.

**Yield:** 12 servings

**Time:** 1 hour

## Ingredients

**Crust**

150 g (¾ cup) granulated sugar

25 g (¼ cup) castor sugar

320 g (2 ½ cups) all-purpose flour

225 g (1 cup) butter, room-temperature and cubed

1 tsp vanilla extract

**Filling**

400 g (2 cups) castor sugar

6 large eggs

Zest of 1 lemon

120 mL (½ cup) lemon juice

**Garnish**

50 g (½ cup) desiccated coconut

## Method

1. Preheat the oven to 180°C (350°F).

2. Combine the sugars and flour for the crust in a large bowl or food processor.

3. Once combined, add the butter and vanilla and mix, either in the food processor or with an electric hand mixer.

4. Line a 23x33 cm (9x13 inch) baking dish with baking paper (or grease it with butter).

5. Place the crust mixture into the pan and press firmly to make sure there aren't any gaps or holes in the crust.

6. Blind bake (prebake) the crust for 15 to 20 minutes or until slightly golden.

7. While the crust is baking, make the filling mixture by combining the sugar, eggs, lemon zest, and lemon juice.

8. When the crust is done, pour the filling mixture into the crust.

9. Bake for another 30 to 35 minutes or until the centre no longer wiggles.

10. Remove from the oven and let cool before sprinkling with the desiccated coconut.

11. Let the bars cool completely before slicing.

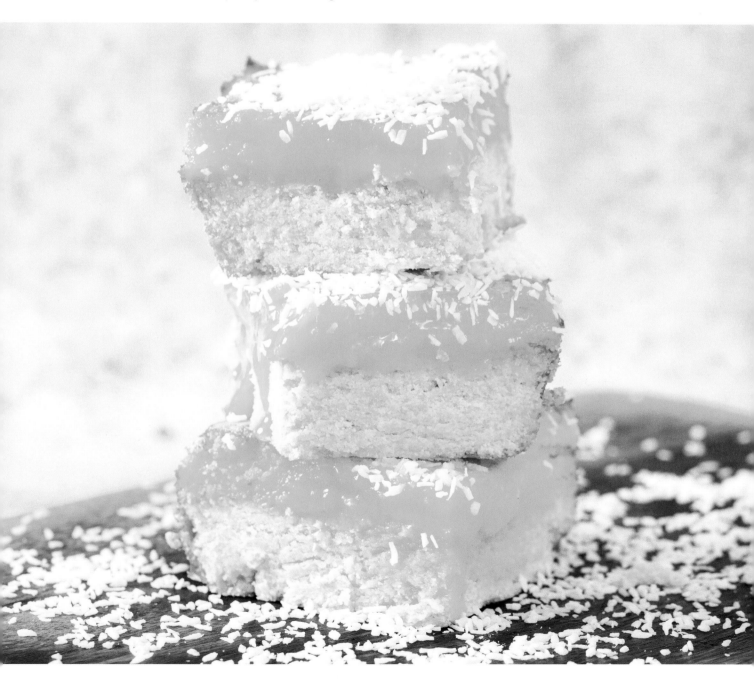

# Brown-Butter Cookies

You know those soft and chewy cookies you remember eating as a child? These are better. Fights have broken out over these during recipe testing, so beware . . .

## Ingredients

285 g (1 ¼ cups) butter

105 g (½ cup) castor sugar

215 g (1 cup) brown sugar

1 medium egg

1 teaspoon vanilla

328 g (2 ½ cups) white or wholemeal flour

1 tsp baking powder

½ teaspoon salt

425 g (2 ½ cups) chocolate chips (We mixed white and milk choc chips.)

## Method

1. Melt the butter in a saucepan over medium-high heat until it starts to turn golden. Pour into your mixing bowl.

2. Let the butter cool in the fridge until it's a room-temperature consistency—you want your butter to be solid. (If you use it when it's still liquid, your cookies will be flat.)

3. Preheat oven to 180°C (350°F) and line a baking tray with baking paper.

4. Once the butter has set, cream together butter, both sugars, egg, and vanilla for 2 to 3 minutes until the mixture is pale and fluffy.

5. Add in the flour, baking powder, and salt until combined—overmixing will make the cookies tough.

6. Stir in the chocolate chips.

7. Take ¼ cup of dough and shape into round balls.

8. Bake 8 to 10 minutes, until the top and edges are just golden.

9. Cool cookies on baking sheet for 2 to 3 minutes before moving to a cooling rack.

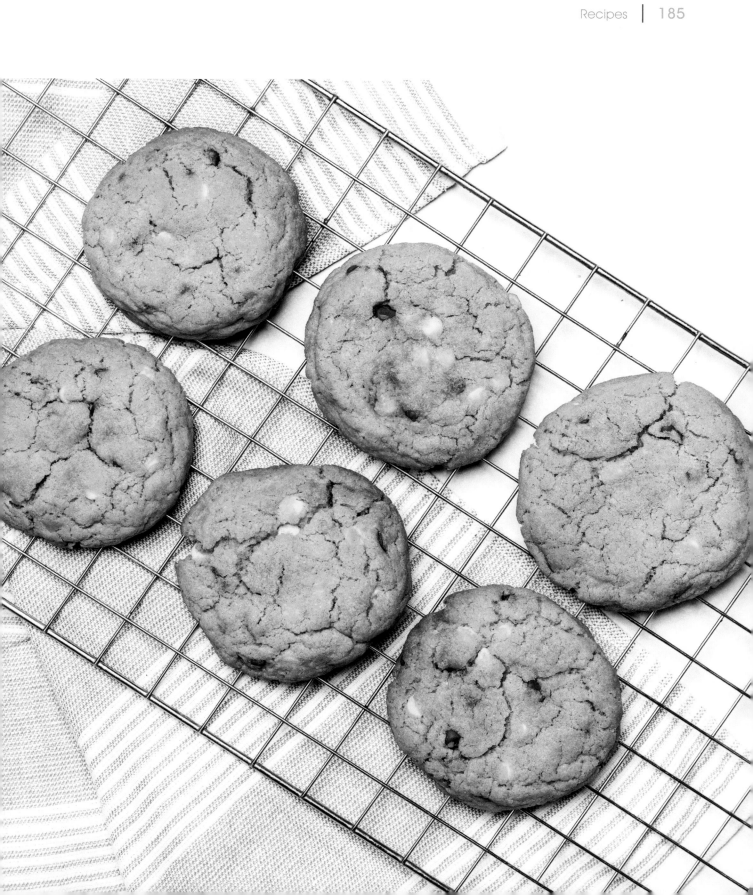

# Trail-Mix Bark

This is one of our favourite recipes in the whole book. The tastes and textures work so well together, and it's perfect for keeping in the fridge for snacking on or as a post-dinner treat.

**Yield:** 8 to 10 servings

## Ingredients

400 g (4 large bars) dark chocolate

60 mL (¼ cup) coconut oil

75 g (1 cup) mini pretzels

60 g (½ cup) dried cranberries

100 g (⅔ cup) chopped mixed nuts

## Method

1. Break up the chocolate into a saucepan and melt over medium heat.

2. Once melted, stir in the coconut oil.

3. Break up the mini pretzels (you can also leave some whole) and add them, along with the cranberries and mixed nuts, to the chocolate.

4. Line a 20x20 cm (8x8 inch) baking tray with baking paper and pour the chocolate mix into the tray.

5. Let it set in the fridge for at least 2 hours.

6. Break up and enjoy!

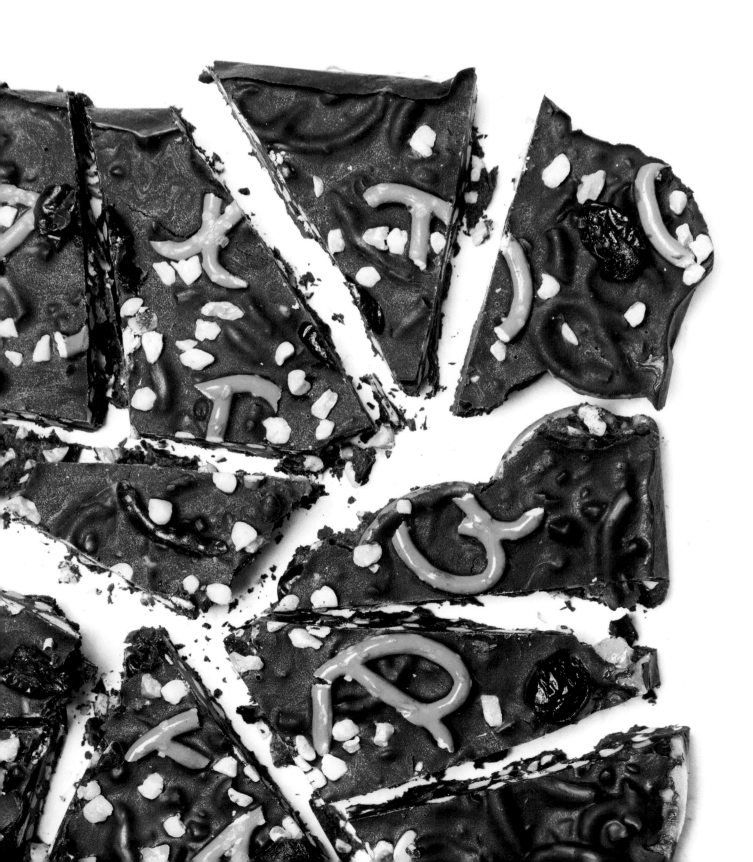

# Peanut-Butter Jam Bread

We feel the PB-and-jam combo is a bit like marmite—you either love it or hate it. You guessed it—we love it, and if you're not keen, maybe this recipe will convert you.

**Time:** 55 minutes

Ingredients

170 g (1 ½ cups) spelt flour

150 g (¾ cup) brown sugar

1 tsp of baking powder

1 egg

250 mL (1 cup) plant-based milk

1 tsp vanilla extract

1 medium banana, mashed

120 g (½ cup) peanut butter

160 g (½ cup) strawberry jam

Extra peanut butter

Extra strawberry jam

Handful of freeze-dried raspberries (optional)

Method

1. Preheat the oven to 180°C (350°F) and line a 450 g (1 lb) loaf tin with baking paper.

2. In a bowl, mix together the flour, sugar, and baking powder.

3. Add the egg, milk, vanilla extract, and mashed banana.

4. Mix well and stir in the 120 g peanut butter and 160 g jam.

5. Pour the mixture into the prepared tin.

6. Bake for 50 minutes, until golden on the outside, then remove from the oven.

7. Allow to cool and add more peanut butter and jam.

8. Top with freeze-dried raspberries if desired.

9. Slice up and enjoy!

# Snacks and Sides

## Bliss Balls

These are great snacks to keep in the fridge or even freeze.

**Time:** 35 minutes

### Ingredients

100 g (¾ cup) fresh raspberries

175 g (1 ¼ cups) dates, chopped

100 g (1 cup) oats

25 g (¼ cup) ground almonds

1 tbsp melted coconut oil

75 g (¾ cup) desiccated coconut, *divided*

### Method

1.  Place the raspberries, dates, oats, ground almonds, coconut oil, and half of the coconut in a food processor.

2.  Blend until well combined.

3.  Wet your hands and roll the mixture into balls.

4.  Place the rest of the desiccated coconut in a shallow bowl and roll each bliss ball around until it's covered.

5.  Place on baking paper on a baking tray and let set in the fridge for 30 minutes.

# Pickled Red Onions

These are the perfect topper to any burrito bowl, tacos, or egg dish. These also go great with the Quinoa Greek Salad With Falafels (see recipe index).

**Time:** 24 hours

## Ingredients

1 red onion, sliced thin

1 tbsp sugar

240 mL (1 cup) white vinegar

## Method

1. Place the sliced red onion, sugar, and vinegar into a jar.

2. Fill the remaining space with water.

3. Seal the jar and place in the fridge for 24 hours.

# Avocado Parm Crisps

Avocado with cheese and seasoning, baked in the oven—need we say more?

**Time:** 20 minutes

## Ingredients

1 large ripe avocado, peeled, pitted, and mashed

½ tsp garlic powder

½ tsp dried basil

½ tsp dried parsley

75 g (¾ cup) parmesan cheese, finely grated

1 ½ tsp lemon juice

Salt and cracked black pepper to taste

## Method

1. Preheat the oven to 180°C (350°F).

2. Combine all the ingredients into a medium-sized bowl.

3. Line a baking tray with baking paper and scoop a tablespoon-sized amount onto the tray.

4. Flatten it out and repeat, leaving a few centimetres between each crisp.

5. Bake for 30 minutes and let them cool completely before serving.

# Sweet-Potato Chips

These sweet-potato chips (fries) are the ultimate side dish. We believe that the tastiest way to enjoy sweet potatoes is in the form of homemade chips.

**Yield:** 2 servings

Time 40 minutes

## Ingredients

2 medium sweet potatoes

2 tbsp avocado oil or olive oil

½ tsp garlic powder

Salt and cracked black pepper to taste

## Method

1. Preheat the oven to 180°C (350°F) and slice the sweet potatoes into long slices approximately ½ cm (¼ inch) thick.

2. Place them on a baking tray and drizzle with avocado oil.

3. Use your hands to toss them around so each is covered, then season with garlic powder, salt, and pepper.

4. Shake the tray to spread the seasoning.

5. Baking in the oven for 30 to 40 minutes, tossing halfway through.

# Halloumi Chips

The only thing better than chips are halloumi chips!

**Yield:** 2 servings

**Time:** 20 minutes

## Ingredients

225 g (1 block) halloumi

½ tsp paprika

3 tbsp plain flour

Olive oil

Dipping sauce of your choice

## Method

1. Cut the halloumi into even-sized chips (fries).

2. Mix the paprika with the flour and cover each halloumi chip.

3. Heat some olive oil in a large pan over medium-heat and cook the chips until golden on each side.

4. Serve with your favourite dipping sauce.

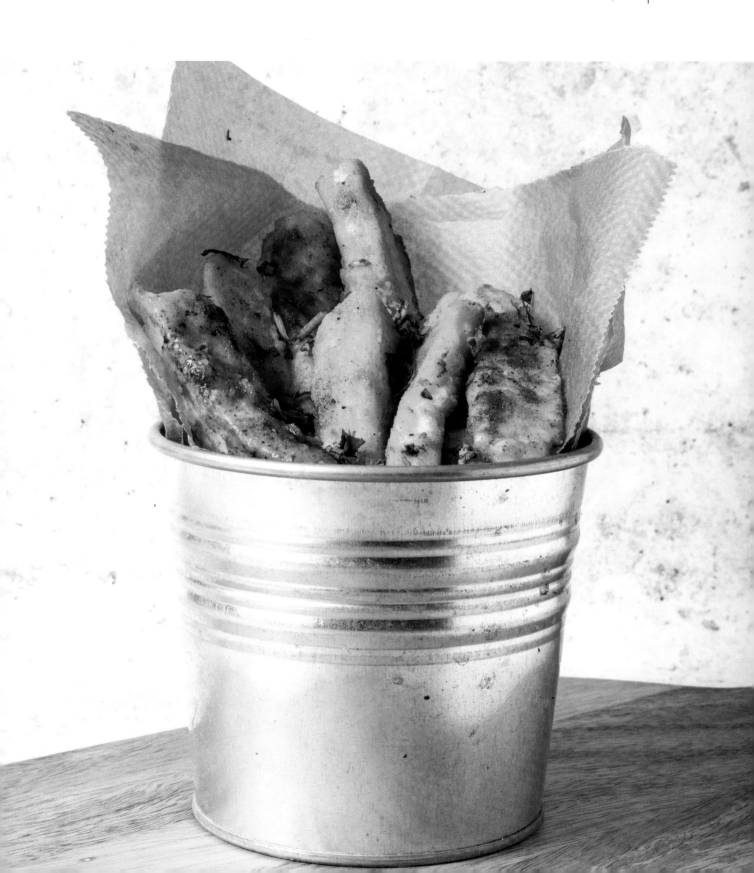

# Sun-Dried Tomato Pesto

This pesto is best served with pasta, spread on toast, or even mixed in with hummus—yum!

**Time:** 15 minutes

## Ingredients

2 large cloves garlic

65 g (½ cup) pine nuts

50 g (1 cup) sun-dried tomatoes

1 tbsp fresh rosemary leaves

10 g (½ cup) fresh basil, tightly packed

½ tsp salt

¼ tsp cracked black pepper

150 mL (⅔ cup) extra-virgin olive oil

## Method

1. In a food processor, start by adding the whole cloves of garlic and pulse until minced.

2. Add the remaining ingredients except for the extra-virgin olive oil and pulse until smooth.

3. Drizzle in the extra-virgin olive oil making sure it's incorporated evenly. Scrape the sides to make sure everything is mixed well.

4. Adjust the seasonings if necessary.

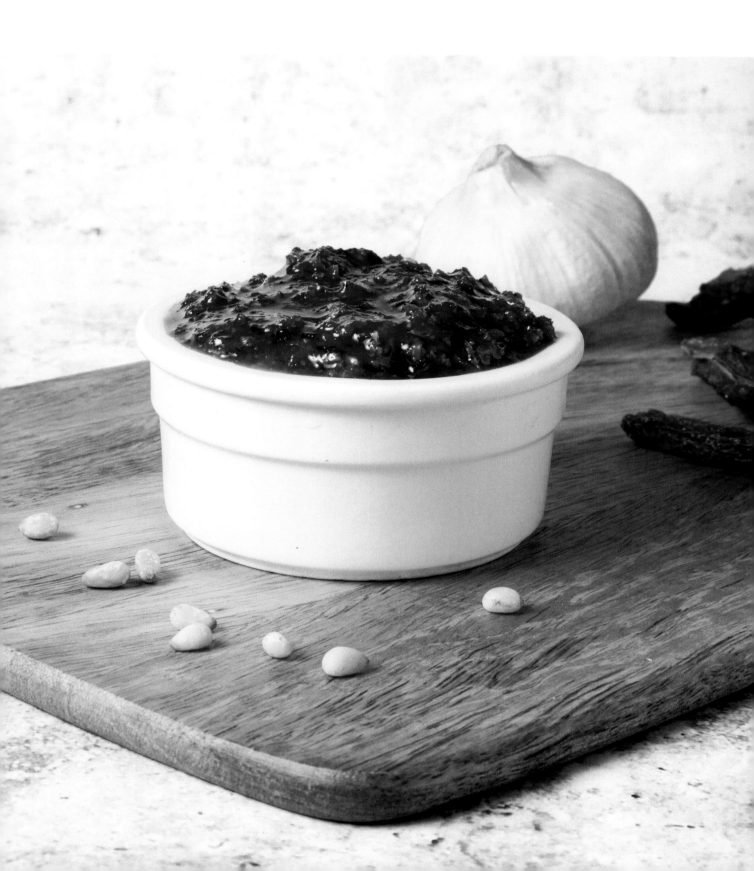

# Classic Basil Pesto

What's a recipe book without classic pesto?

**Time:** 15 minutes

## Ingredients

2 large cloves garlic

30g (¼ cup) pine nuts

15 g (¼ cup) nutritional yeast

40 g (2 cups) basil

1 tsp lemon zest

1 tsp lemon juice

½ tsp salt

¼ tsp black pepper

150 mL extra-virgin olive oil

## Method

1. In a food processor, start by adding the whole cloves of garlic and pulse until minced.

2. Add the remaining ingredients except for the extra-virgin olive oil and pulse until smooth.

3. Drizzle in the extra-virgin olive oil making sure it's incorporated evenly. Scrape the sides to make sure everything is mixed well.

4. Adjust the seasonings if necessary.

# Peanut Dressing

Peanut butter makes everything better. That's a fact. No, we don't have a research study to back that up, but trust us.

**Time:** 15 minutes

Ingredients:

2 tbsp smooth peanut butter (or tahini if allergic to peanuts)

2 tbsp extra-virgin olive oil

2 tbsp soya sauce

2 tsp fresh garlic, minced

1 ½ tbsp rice wine vinegar

½ tsp cold-pressed sesame oil

2 tsp maple syrup

2 tbsp spring onions (scallions), sliced thin

1 tsp red pepper flakes

Water as needed

Method

1. Combine all ingredients in a small mixing bowl.

2. Thin with water until desired consistency.

# Avocado-and-Coriander Dip

Bari's mum, Franny, calls this 'crack sauce'. We think she means it's addictive.

**Time:** 10 minutes

## Ingredients

1 ripe avocado, peeled and pitted

Juice of 1 large lime

50 g (1 cup) coriander (cilantro), packed tightly

Salt and cracked black pepper to taste

Water

## Method

1.  Combine the avocado, lime juice, coriander, salt, and pepper into a food processor or blender.

2.  Blitz.

3.  Add water until the sauce is the desired consistency and adjust seasoning to taste.

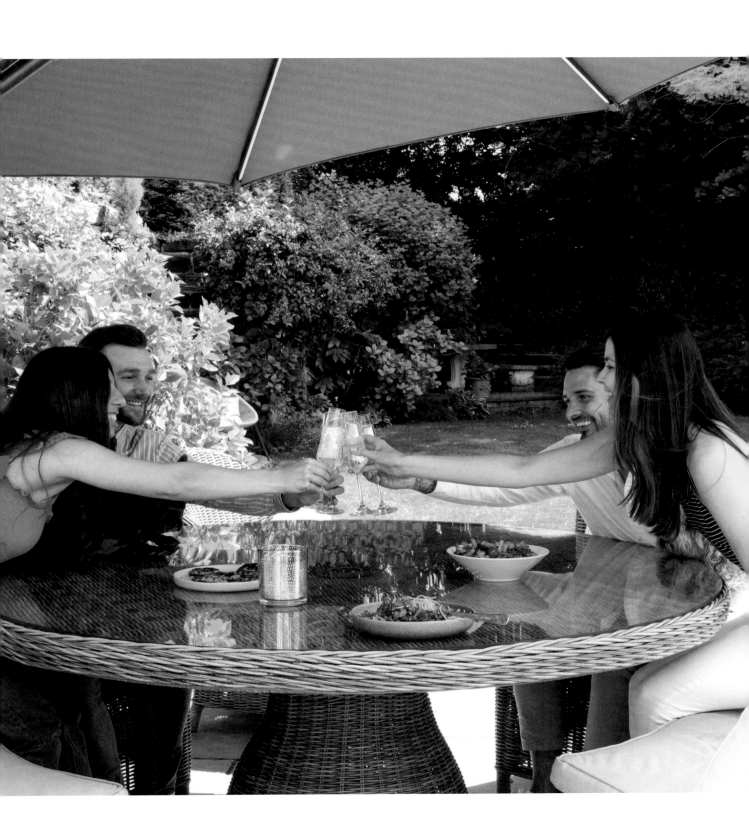

# References

Albers, S. 2009. *Eating Mindfully: How to End Mindless Eating and Enjoy a Balanced Relationship With Food.* Read How You Want, Limited. https://books.google.co.uk/books?id=RKPJmGk1tf0C.

Almeida, O. P., A. H. Ford, V. Hirani, V. Singh, F. M. vanBockxmeer, K. McCaul, and L. Flicker. 2014. 'B Vitamins to Enhance Treatment Response to Antidepressants in Middle-aged and Older Adults: Results From the B-VITAGE Randomised, Double-Blind, Placebo-Controlled Trial'. *British Journal of Psychiatry* 205, no. 6 (December): 450–57. https://doi.org/10.1192/bjp.bp.114.145177.

Ambwani, S., M. Shippe, Z. Gao, and S. B. Austin. 2019. 'Is #Cleaneating a Healthy or Harmful Dietary Strategy? Perceptions of Clean Eating and Associations With Disordered Eating Among Young Adults'. *Journal of Eating Disorders 7*, no. 17 (June). https://doi.org/10.1186/s40337-019-0246-2.

American Heart Association. 2018. 'Healthy Cooking Oils'. Heart.org. Last Reviewed April 24, 2018. https://www.heart.org/en/healthy-living/healthy-eating/eat-smart/fats/healthy-cooking-oils.

Anderson, D. E., and M. S. Hickey. 1994. 'Effects of Caffeine on the Metabolic and Catecholamine Responses to Exercise in 5 and 28 Degrees C'. *Medicine and Science in Sports and Exercise* 26, no. 4 (April): 453–58.

Anderson, E., and G. Shivakumar. 2013. 'Effects of Exercise and Physical Activity on Anxiety'. *Frontiers in Psychiatry* 4, no. 27 (April). https://doi.org/10.3389/fpsyt.2013.00027.

Anderson, L. A., and J. B. Gross. 2004. 'Aromatherapy With Peppermint, Isopropyl Alcohol, or Placebo Is Equally Effective in Relieving Postoperative Nausea'. *Journal of PeriAnesthesia Nursing* 19, no. 1 (February): 29–35. https://doi.org/10.1016/j.jopan.2003.11.001.

Archer, E., G. Pavela, and C. J. Lavie. 2015. 'The Inadmissibility of What We Eat in America and NHANES Dietary Data in Nutrition and Obesity Research and the Scientific Formulation of National Dietary Guidelines'. *Mayo Clinic Proceedings* 90, no. 7 (July): 911–26. https://doi.org/10.1016/j.mayocp.2015.04.009.

Arens, U. 2020. 'Food Fact Sheet: Food and Mood'. The British Dietetic Association (BDA). Last reviewed August 2020. https://www.bda.uk.com/uploads/assets/2f4bf991-0aaf-4d2c-8a56067a2055d9d7/Food-and-Mood-food-fact-sheet.pdf.

Ascherio, A., M. G. Weisskopf, E. J. O'Reilly, M. L. McCullough, E. E. Calle, C. Rodriguez, and M. J. Thun. 2004. 'Coffee Consumption, Gender, and Parkinson's Disease Mortality in the Cancer Prevention Study II Cohort: The Modifying Effects of Estrogen'. *American Journal of Epidemiology* 160, no. 10 (November): 977–84. https://doi.org/10.1093/aje/kwh312.

Atkins. n.d. 'Phase 1 Frequently Asked Questions & Facts'. How It Works. Accessed [February] [25], [2020]. https://www.atkins.com/how-it-works/atkins-20/phase-1/faq.

Baker, D., and N. Keramidas. 2013. 'The Psychology of Hunger'. *Monitor on Psychology* 44, no. 9 (October): 66.

Barclay, L. R. C., M. R. Vinqvist, K. Mukai, H. Goto, Y. Hashimoto, A. Tokunaga, and H. Uno. 2000. 'On the Antioxidant Mechanism of Curcumin: Classical Methods Are Needed to Determine Antioxidant Mechanism and Activity'. *Organic Letters* 2, no. 18 (August): 2841–43. https://doi.org/10.1021/ol000173t.

Barney, J. L., H. B. Murray, S. M. Manasse, C. Dochat, and A. S. Juarascio. 2019. 'Mechanisms and Moderators in Mindfulness- and Acceptance-Based Treatments for Binge Eating Spectrum Disorders: A Systematic Review'. *European Eating Disorders Review* 27, no. 4 (July): 352–80. https://doi.org/10.1002/erv.2673.

BDA (The British Dietetic Association). 2019. 'One Blue Dot—the BDA's Environmentally Sustainable Diet Project'. Resource Library. July 2019. https://www.bda.uk.com/resource/one-blue-dot.html.

Benabou, R., and J. Tirole. 2003. 'Intrinsic and Extrinsic Motivation'. Review of Economic Studies 70, no. 3 (July): 489–520. https://econpapers.repec.org/RePEc:oup:restud:v:70:y:2003:i:3:p:489-520.

Berger, M., J. A. Gray, and B. L. Roth. 2009. 'The Expanded Biology of Serotonin'. *Annual Review of Medicine* 60 (February): 355–66. https://doi.org/10.1146/annurev.med.60.042307.110802.

Black, C. D., M. P. Herring, D. J. Hurley, and P. J. O'Connor. 2010. 'Ginger (*Zingiber officinale*) Reduces Muscle Pain Caused by Eccentric Exercise'. *Journal of Pain* 11, no. 9 (September): 894–903. https://doi.org/10.1016/j.jpain.2009.12.013.

Bonardi, J. M. T., L. G. Lima, G. O. Campos, R. F. Bertani, J. C. Moriguti, E. Ferriolli, and N. K. C. Lima. 2016. 'Effect of Different Types of Exercise on Sleep Quality of Elderly Subjects'. Sleep Medicine 25 (September): 122–29. https://doi.org/10.1016/j.sleep.2016.06.025.

Booth, F. W., C. K. Roberts, and M. J. Laye. 2012. 'Lack of Exercise Is a Major Cause of Chronic Diseases'. *Comprehensive Physiology* 2, no. 2 (April): 1143–211. https://doi.org/10.1002/cphy.c110025.

Boskey, A. L., and R. Coleman. 2010. 'Aging and Bone'. *Journal of Dental Research*, 89, no. 12 (October): 1333–48. https://doi.org/10.1177/0022034510377791.

Bourassa, M. W., I. Alim, S. J. Bultman, and R. R. Ratan. 2016. 'Butyrate, Neuroepigenetics and the Gut Microbiome: Can a High Fiber Diet Improve Brain Health?' *Neuroscience Letters* 625 (June): 56–63. https://doi.org/10.1016/j.neulet.2016.02.009.

Brownley, K. A., N. D. Berkman, C. M. Peat, K. N. Lohr, K. E. Cullen, C. M. Bann, and C. M. Bulik. 2016. 'Binge-Eating Disorder in Adults: A Systematic Review and Meta-analysis'. *Annals of Internal Medicine* 165, no. 6 (September): 409–20. https://doi.org/10.7326/M15-2455.

Bruce, L. J., and L. A. Ricciardelli. 2016. 'A Systematic Review of the Psychosocial Correlates of Intuitive Eating Among Adult Women'. *Appetite* 96 (January): 454–72. https://doi.org/10.1016/j.appet.2015.10.012.

Buford, T. W., and D. S. Willoughby. 2008. 'Impact of DHEA(S) and Cortisol on Immune Function in Aging: A Brief Review'. *Applied Physiology, Nutrition, and Metabolism* no. 3 (April): 429–33. https://doi.org/10.1139/H08-013.

Burton, A. L., and M. J. Abbott. 2019. 'Processes and Pathways to Binge Eating: Development of an Integrated Cognitive and Behavioural Model of Binge Eating'. *Journal of Eating Disorders* 7, no. 18 (June). https://doi.org/10.1186/s40337-019-0248-0.

Castillo-Fernandez, J. E., T. D. Spector, and J. T. Bell. 2014. 'Epigenetics of Discordant Monozygotic Twins: Implications for Disease'. *Genome Medicine* 6, no. 60 (July). https://doi.org/10.1186/s13073-014-0060-z.

Chandran, B., and A. Goel. 2012. 'A Randomized, Pilot Study to Assess the Efficacy and Safety of Curcumin in Patients With Active Rheumatoid Arthritis'. *Phytotherapy Research* 26, no. 11 (November): 1719–25. https://doi.org/10.1002/ptr.4639.

Cheuvront, S. N. 2003. 'The Zone Diet Phenomenon: A Closer Look at the Science Behind the Claims'. Journal of the *American College of Nutrition* 22 (1): 9–17. https://doi.org/10.1080/07315724.2003.10719271.

Cian, C., P. A. Barraud, B. Melin, and C. Raphel. 2001. 'Effects of Fluid Ingestion on Cognitive Function After Heat Stress or Exercise-Induced Dehydration'. *International Journal of Psychophysiology* 42, no. 3 (November): 243–51. https://doi.org/10.1016/s0167-8760(01)00142-8.

Clear, J. 2018. *Atomic Habits: An Easy & Proven Way to Build Good Habits & Break Bad Ones*. New York: Avery.

Cookie Diet. n.d. 'History of the Real Dr. Siegal's Cookie Diet'. About Us. Accessed [January] [27], [2020 https://www.cookiediet.com/about-us/cookie-history/.

Cotman, C. W., N. C. Berchtold, and L. Christie. 2007. 'Exercise Builds Brain Health: Key Roles of Growth Factor Cascades and Inflammation'. *Trends in Neurosciences* 30, no. 9 (September): 464–72. https://doi.org/10.1016/j.tins.2007.06.011.

Cummings, D. E., J. Q. Purnell, R. S. Frayo, K. Schmidova, B. E. Wisse, and D. S. Weigle. 2001. 'A Preprandial Rise in Plasma Ghrelin Levels Suggests a Role in Meal Initiation in Humans'. *Diabetes* 50, no. 8 (August): 1714–19. https://doi.org/10.2337/diabetes.50.8.1714.

Davidson, L. S. 2013. 'Subway Diet'. MSN. January 1, 2013. https://www.msn.com/en-us/news/other/subway-diet/ar-AA8mPo.

de Menezes, E. V. A., H. A. d. C. Sampaio, A. A. F. Carioca, N. A. Parente, F. O. Brito, T. M. M. Moreira, A. C. C. de Souza, and S. P. M. Arruda. 2019. 'Influence of Paleolithic Diet on Anthropometric Markers in Chronic Diseases: Systematic Review and Meta-analysis'. *Nutrition Journal* 18, no. 41 (July). https://doi.org/10.1186/s12937-019-0457-z.

de Wit, S., M. Kindt, S. L. Knot, A. A. C. Verhoeven, T. W. Robbins, J. Gasull-Camos, M. Evans, H. Mirza, and C. M. Gillan. 2018. 'Shifting the Balance Between Goals and Habits: Five Failures in Experimental Habit Induction'. *Journal of Experimental Psychology: General* 147, no. 7 (July): 1043–65. https://doi.org/10.1037/xge0000402.

Di Milia, L., C. Vandelanotte, and M. J. Duncan. 2013. 'The Association Between Short Sleep and Obesity After Controlling for Demographic, Lifestyle, Work and Health Related Factors'. *Sleep Medicine* 14, no. 4 (April): 319–23. https://doi.org/10.1016/j.sleep.2012.12.007.

Doherty, M., and P. M. Smith. 2004. 'Effects of Caffeine Ingestion on Exercise Testing: A Meta-analysis'. *International Journal of Sport Nutrition and Exercise Metabolism* 14, no. 6 (December): 626–46. https://doi.org/10.1123/ijsnem.14.6.626.

———. 2005. 'Effects of Caffeine Ingestion on Rating of Perceived Exertion During and After Exercise: A Meta-analysis'. *Scandinavian Journal of Medicine & Science in Sports* 15, no. 2 (April): 69–78. https://doi.org/10.1111/j.1600-0838.2005.00445.x.

Donini, L. M., D. Marsili, M. P. Graziani, M. Ibriale, and C. Canella. 2005. 'Orthorexia Nervosa: Validation of a Diagnosis Questionnaire'. *Eating and Weight Disorders* 10, no. 2 (June): e28-e32.

Donovan, L. 2018. 'Food Fact Sheet: Fats'. The British Dietetic Association (BDA). January 2018. https://www.bda.uk.com/uploads/assets/84f584f6-9294-4a5f-8012bf20e7bedd56/Fat-food-fact-sheet.pdf.

Driver, H. S., and S. R. Taylor. 2000. 'Exercise and Sleep'. *Sleep Medicine Reviews* 4, no. 4 (August): 387–402. https://doi.org/10.1053/smrv.2000.0110.

Duhigg, C. 2014. *The Power of Habit: Why We Do What We Do in Life and Business*. New York: Random House Trade Paperbacks. 2014. https://search.library.wisc.edu/catalog/9910195246302121.

Dunn, T. M., and S. Bratman. 2016. 'On Orthorexia Nervosa: A Review of the Literature and Proposed Diagnostic Criteria'. *Eating Behaviors* 21 (April): 11–17. https://doi.org/10.1016/j.eatbeh.2015.12.006.

Durlach, J., N. Pages, P. Bac, M. Bara, and A. Guiet-Bara. 2002. 'Biorhythms and Possible Central Regulation of Magnesium Status, Phototherapy, Darkness Therapy and Chronopathological Forms of Magnesium Depletion'. *Magnesium Research* 15, no. 1–2 (March): 49–66.

Duscha, B. D., C. A. Slentz, J. L. Johnson, J. A. Houmard, D. R. Bensimhon, K. J. Knetzger, and W. E. Kraus. 2005. 'Effects of Exercise Training Amount and Intensity on Peak Oxygen Consumption in Middle-Age Men and Women at Risk for Cardiovascular Disease'. *CHEST* 128, no. 4 (October): 2788–93. https://doi.org/10.1378/chest.128.4.2788.

El-Baroty, G. S., H. H. Abd El-Baky, R. S. Farag, and M. A. Saleh. 2010. 'Characterization of Antioxidant and Antimicrobial Compounds of Cinnamon and Ginger Essential Oils'. *African Journal of Biochemistry Research* 4, no. 6 (June): 167–174.

Ellenbogen, J. M. 2005. 'Cognitive Benefits of Sleep and Their Loss Due to Sleep Deprivation'. *Neurology* 64, no. 7 (April): E25–E27. https://doi.org/10.1212/01.wnl.0000164850.68115.81.

Ernst, E., and M. H. Pittler. 2000. 'Efficacy of Ginger for Nausea and Vomiting: A Systematic Review of Randomized Clinical Trials'. *British Journal of Anaesthesia* 84, no. 3 (March): 367–71. https://doi.org/10.1093/oxfordjournals.bja.a013442.

Esfahani, A., J. M. W. Wong, J. Truan, C. R. Villa, A. Mirrahimi, K. Srichaikul, and C. W. C. Kendall. 2011. 'Health Effects of Mixed Fruit and Vegetable Concentrates: A Systematic Review of the Clinical Interventions'. *Journal of the American College of Nutrition* 30 (5): 285–294. https://doi.org/10.1080/07315724.2011.10719971.

Esposito, K., M. I. Maiorino, G. Bellastella, P. Chiodini, D. Panagiotakos, and D. Giugliano. 2015. 'A Journey Into a Mediterranean Diet and Type 2 Diabetes: A Systematic Review With Meta-analyses'. *BMJ Open* 5, no. 8 (August): e008222. https://doi.org/10.1136/bmjopen-2015-008222.

F-Factor. n.d. *'What Is F-Factor?'* F-Factor. Accessed [February] [25], [2020]. https://www.ffactor.com/what-is-f-factor/.

Fenton, T. R., and C. J. Fenton. 2016. 'Paleo Diet Still Lacks Evidence'. *American Journal of Clinical Nutrition* 104, no. 3 (September): 844. https://doi.org/10.3945/ajcn.116.139006.

Fenton, T. R., A. W. Lyon, M. Eliasziw, S. C. Tough, and D. A. Hanley. 2009. 'Phosphate Decreases Urine Calcium and Increases Calcium Balance: A Meta-analysis of the Osteoporosis Acid-Ash Diet Hypothesis'. *Nutrition Journal* 8, no. 41 (September). https://doi.org/10.1186/1475-2891-8-41.

Field, T., M. Hernandez-Reif, M. Diego, S. Schanberg, and C. Kuhn. 2005. 'Cortisol Decreases and Serotonin and Dopamine Increase Following Massage Therapy'. *International Journal of Neuroscience* 115, no. 10 (October): 1397–413. https://doi.org/10.1080/00207450590956459.

Ford, A. C., N. J. Talley, B. M. R. Spiegel, A. E. Foxx-Orenstein, L. Schiller, E. M. M. Quigley, and P. Moayyedi. 2008. 'Effect of Fibre, Antispasmodics, and Peppermint Oil in the Treatment of Irritable Bowel Syndrome: Systematic Review and Meta-analysis'. *BMJ* 337, no. 7683 (December): a2313. https://doi.org/10.1136/bmj.a2313.

Frey, R. J. n.d. 'Cabbage Soup Diet'. reference.jrank.org/diets. Accessed [January] [27], [2020]. https://reference.jrank.org/diets/Cabbage_Soup_Diet.html.

Gaffney-Stomberg, E., K. L. Insogna, N. R. Rodriguez, and J. E. Kerstetter. 2009. 'Increasing Dietary Protein Requirements in Elderly People for Optimal Muscle and Bone Health'. *Journal of the American Geriatrics Society* 57, no. 6 (June): 1073–79. https://doi.org/10.1111/j.1532-5415.2009.02285.x.

Galbete, C., L. Schwingshackl, C. Schwedhelm, H. Boeing, and M. B. Schulze. 2018. 'Evaluating Mediterranean Diet and Risk of Chronic Disease in Cohort Studies: An Umbrella Review of Meta-analyses'. *European Journal of Epidemiology* 33, no. 10 (October): 909–31. https://doi.org/10.1007/s10654-018-0427-3.

Gardner, B., P. Lally, and J. Wardle. 2012. 'Making Health Habitual: The Psychology of "Habit-Formation" and General Practice'. *British Journal of General Practice* 62, no. 605 (December): 664–66. https://doi.org/10.3399/bjgp12X659466.

Gardner, C. D., A. Kiazand, S. Alhassan, S. Kim, R. S. Stafford, R. R. Balise, H. C. Kraemer, and A. C. King. 2007. 'Comparison of the Atkins, Zone, Ornish, and LEARN Diets for Change in Weight and Related Risk Factors Among Overweight Premenopausal Women: The A to Z Weight Loss Study: A Randomized Trial'. *JAMA* 297, no. 9 (March): 969–77. https://doi.org/10.1001/jama.297.9.969.

Gilbert, S. S., C. J. van den Heuvel, S. A. Ferguson, and D. Dawson. 2004. 'Thermoregulation as a Sleep Signalling System'. *Sleep Medicine Reviews* 8, no 2 (April): 81–93. https://doi.org/10.1016/S1087-0792(03)00023-6.

Godos, J., R. Ferri, F. Caraci, F. I. I. Cosentino, S. Castellano, F. Galvano, and G. Grosso. 2019. 'Adherence to the Mediterranean Diet is Associated With Better Sleep Quality in Italian Adults'. *Nutrients* 11, no. 5 (April): 976. https://doi.org/10.3390/nu11050976.

Goldman, S. E., K. L. Stone, S. Ancoli-Israel, T. Blackwell, S. K. Ewing, R. Boudreau, J. A. Cauley, M. Hall, K. A. Matthews, and A. B. Newman. 2007. 'Poor Sleep Is Associated With Poorer Physical Performance and Greater Functional Limitations in Older Women'. *Sleep* 30, no. 10 (October): 1317–24. https://doi.org/10.1093/sleep/30.10.1317.

Goswami, J. N., and S. Sharma. 2019. 'Current Perspectives on the Role of the Ketogenic Diet in Epilepsy Management'. *Neuropsychiatric Disease and Treatment* 15 (November): 3273–85. https://doi.org/10.2147/NDT.S201862.

Gow, M. L., M. Ho, T. L. Burrows, L. A. Baur, L. Stewart, M. J. Hutchesson, C. T. Cowell, C. E. Collins, and S. P. Garnett. 2014. 'Impact of Dietary Macronutrient Distribution on BMI and Cardiometabolic Outcomes in Overweight and Obese Children and Adolescents: A Systematic Review'. *Nutrition Reviews* 72, no. 7 (July): 453–70. https://doi.org/10.1111/nure.12111.

Grossman, P., L. Niemann, S. Schmidt, and H. Walach. 2004. 'Mindfulness-Based Stress Reduction and Health Benefits: A Meta-analysis'. *Journal of Psychosomatic Research* 57, no. 1 (July): 35–43. https://doi.org/10.1016/S0022-3999(03)00573-7.

Halbert, J. A., C. A. Silagy, P. Finucane, R. T. Withers, P. A. Hamdorf, and G. R. Andrews. 1997. 'The Effectiveness of Exercise Training in Lowering Blood Pressure: A Meta-analysis of Randomised Controlled Trials of 4 Weeks or Longer'. *Journal of Human Hypertension* 11, no. 10 (October): 641–49. https://doi.org/10.1038/sj.jhh.1000509.

Harper, A., T. Larsen, and A. Astrup. (2004) 2005. 'Atkins and Other Low-Carbohydrate Diets: Hoax or an Effective Tool for Weight Loss?'. *Lancet 364*, no. 9437 (September): 897–99. Secondary publication, *Ugeskrift for Læger* 167, no. 10 (March) 1183–85. Citations refer to the Ugeskrift publication.

Harvard T. H. Chan School of Public Health. n.d. 'Fiber'. The Nutrition Source. Accessed [Januray] [15], [2020]. https://www.hsph.harvard.edu/nutritionsource/carbohydrates/fiber/.

Herman, C. P., and D. Mack. 1975. 'Restrained and Unrestrained Eating'. *Journal of Personality* 43, no. 4 (December): 647–60. https://doi.org/10.1111/j.1467-6494.1975.tb00727.x.

Hirotsu, C., S. Tufik, and M. L. Andersen. 2015. Interactions Between Sleep, Stress, and Metabolism: From Physiological to Pathological Conditions. *Sleep Science* 8, no. 3 (November): 143–52. https://doi.org/10.1016/j.slsci.2015.09.002.

Huxley, R., C. M. Y. Lee, F. Barzi, L. Timmermeister, S. Czernichow, V. Perkovic, D. E. Grobbee, D. Batty, and M. Woodward. 2009. 'Coffee, Decaffeinated Coffee, and Tea Consumption in Relation to Incident Type 2 Diabetes Mellitus: A Systematic Review With Meta-analysis. *Archives of Internal Medicine* 169, no. 22 (December): 2053–63. https://doi.org/10.1001/archinternmed.2009.439.

Jackson, J., and C. Collins. 2014. 'Food Fact Sheet: Healthy Eating'. The British Dietetic Association (BDA). Last reviewed August 2019. https://www.bda.uk.com/resource/healthy-eating.html.

Jenkins, T. A., J. C. D. Nguyen, K. E. Polglaze, and P. P. Bertrand. 2016. 'Influence of Tryptophan and Serotonin on Mood and Cognition with a Possible Role of the Gut-Brain Axis'. *Nutrients* 8, no. 1 (January): 56. https://doi.org/10.3390/nu8010056.

Josling, P. 2001. Preventing the Common Cold With a Garlic Supplement: A Double-Blind, Placebo-Controlled Survey'. *Advances in Therapy* 18, no. 4 (July): 189–93. https://doi.org/10.1007/bf02850113.

Juliano, L. M., and R. R. Griffiths. 2004. 'A critical Review of Caffeine Withdrawal: Empirical Validation of Symptoms and Signs, Incidence, Severity, and Associated Features'. *Psychopharmacology* 176, no. 1 (September): 1–29. https://doi.org/10.1007/s00213-004-2000-x.

Katterman, S. N., B. M. Kleinman, M. M. Hood, L. M. Nackers, and J. A. Corsica. 2014. 'Mindfulness Meditation as an Intervention for Binge Eating, Emotional Eating, and Weight Loss: A Systematic Review. *Eating Behaviors* 15, no. 2 (April): 197–204. https://doi.org/10.1016/j.eatbeh.2014.01.005.

Kellow, J. n.d. 'The Cost of Dieting'. Weight Loss Resources. Accessed [February] [16], [2020]. https://www.weightlossresources.co.uk/diet/diet-cost.htm.

Khanna, R., J. K. MacDonald, and B. G. Levesque. 2014. 'Peppermint Oil for the Treatment of Irritable Bowel Syndrome: A Systematic Review and Meta-analysis'. *Journal of Clinical Gastroenterology* 48, no. 6 (July): 505–12. https://doi.org/10.1097/MCG.0b013e3182a88357.

Kirk-Sanchez, N. J., and E. L. McGough. 2014. 'Physical Exercise and Cognitive Performance in the Elderly: Current Perspectives'. *Clinical Interventions in Aging* 9:51–62. https://doi.org/10.2147/CIA.S39506.

Kirschbaum, C., T. Klauer, S. H. Filipp, and D. H. Hellhammer. 1995. 'Sex-Specific Effects of Social Support on Cortisol and Subjective Responses to Acute Psychological Stress'. *Psychosomatic Medicine* 57, no. 1 (January–February): 23–31. https://doi.org/10.1097/00006842-199501000-00004.

Klok, M. D., S. Jakobsdottir, and M. L. Drent. 2007. 'The Role of Leptin and Ghrelin in the Regulation of Food Intake and Body Weight in Humans: A Review'. *Obesity Reviews* 8, no. 1 (January): 21–34. https://doi.org/10.1111/j.1467-789X.2006.00270.x.

Kornstein, S. G., J. L. Kunovac, B. K. Herman, and L. Culpepper. 2016. 'Recognizing Binge-Eating Disorder in the Clinical Setting: A Review of the Literature'. *Primary Care Companion for CNS Disorders* 18 (3): e1–e9. https://doi.org/10.4088/PCC.15r01905.

Koven, N. S., and A. W. Abry. 2015. 'The Clinical Basis of Orthorexia Nervosa: Emerging Perspectives'. *Neuropsychiatric Disease and Treatment* 11 (February): 385–94. https://doi.org/10.2147/NDT.S61665.

Kredlow, M. A., M. C. Capozzoli, B. A. Hearon, A. W. Calkins, and M. W. Otto. 2015. 'The Effects of Physical Activity on Sleep: A Meta-analytic Review'. *Journal of Behavioral Medicine* 38, no. 3 (June): 427–49. https://doi.org/10.1007/s10865-015-9617-6.

Kristeller, J. L., and R. Q. Wolever. 2011. 'Mindfulness-Based Eating Awareness Training for Treating Binge Eating Disorder: The Conceptual Foundation'. *Eating Disorders* 19, no. 1 (January–February): 49–61. https://doi.org/10.1080/10640266.2011.533605.

Kruszelnicki, K. S. 2002. 'Autopsy'. ABC Science. October 23 2002. https://www.abc.net.au/science/articles/2002/10/23/689035.htm.

La Berge, A. F. 2008. 'How the Ideology of Low Fat Conquered America'. *Journal of the History of Medicine and Allied Sciences* 63, no. 2 (April): 139–77. https://doi.org/10.1093/jhmas/jrn001.

Larrieu, T., and S. Layé. 2018. 'Food for Mood: Relevance of Nutritional Omega-3 Fatty Acids for Depression and Anxiety'. *Frontiers in Physiology* 9, no. 1047 (August). https://doi.org/10.3389/fphys.2018.01047.

Larun, L., K. G. Brurberg, J. Odgaard-Jensen, and J. R. Price. 2016. 'Exercise Therapy for Chronic Fatigue Syndrome'. *Cochrane Database of Systematic Reviews* 12, no. CD003200 (December). https://doi.org/10.1002/14651858.CD003200.pub6.

Lesser, L. I., C. B. Ebbeling, M. Goozner, D. Wypij, and D. S. Ludwig. 2007. 'Relationship Between Funding Source and Conclusion Among Nutrition-Related Scientific Articles'. *PLOS Medicine* 4, no. 1 (January): e5. https://doi.org/10.1371/journal.pmed.0040005.

Lewer, M., A. Bauer, A. S. Hartmann, and S. Vocks. 2017. 'Different Facets of Body Image Disturbance in Binge Eating Disorder: A Review'. *Nutrients* 9, no. 12 (November): 1294. https://doi.org/10.3390/nu9121294.

Lewis, J. E., E. Tiozzo, A. B. Melillo, S. Leonard, L. Chen, A. Mendez, J. M. Woolger, and J. Konefal. 2013. 'The Effect of Methylated Vitamin B Complex on Depressive and Anxiety Symptoms and Quality of Life in Adults With Depression'. *ISRN Psychiatry* 2013, no. 621453 (January). https://doi.org/10.1155/2013/621453.

Lichtenstein, G. R. 2015. 'The Importance of Sleep'. *Gastroenterology & Hepatology* 11, no. 12 (December): 790. https://pubmed.ncbi.nlm.nih.gov/27134595.

Lindseth, G., and A. Murray. 2016. 'Dietary Macronutrients and Sleep'. *Western Journal of Nursing Research* 38, no. 8 (August): 938–58. https://doi.org/10.1177/0193945916643712.

Loprinzi, P., and B. Cardinal. 2011. 'Association Between Objectively-Measured Physical Activity and Sleep, NHANES 2005–2006'. *Mental Health and Physical Activity* 4, no. 2 (December): 65–69. https://doi.org/10.1016/j.mhpa.2011.08.001.

Maia, L., and A. De Mendonça. 2002. 'Does Caffeine Intake Protect From Alzheimer's Disease?' *European Journal of Neurology* 9, no.4 (July): 377–82. https://doi.org/10.1046/j.1468-1331.2002.00421.x.

Mancini, J. G., K. B. Filion, R. Atallah, and M. J. Eisenberg. 2016. 'Systematic Review of the Mediterranean Diet for Long-Term Weight Loss'. *American Journal of Medicine* 129, no. 4 (April): 407–15.e4. https://doi.org/10.1016/j.amjmed.2015.11.028.

Martini, D. 2019. 'Health Benefits of Mediterranean Diet'. *Nutrients* 11, no. 8 (August): 1802. https://doi.org/10.3390/nu11081802.

Masuda, A., M. Price, and R. D. Latzman. 2012. 'Mindfulness Moderates the Relationship Between Disordered Eating Cognitions and Disordered Eating Behaviors in a Non-Clinical College Sample'. *Journal of Psychopathology and Behavioral Assessment* 34, no. 1 (March): 107–15. https://doi.org/10.1007/s10862-011-9252-7.

Matousek, R. H., P. L. Dobkin, and J. Pruessner. 2010. 'Cortisol as a Marker for Improvement in Mindfulness-Based Stress Reduction'. *Complementary Therapies in Clinical Practice* 16, no. 1 (February): 13–19. https://doi.org/10.1016/j.ctcp.2009.06.004.

Mayo Clinic Staff. 2017. 'Water: How much should you drink Every Day?' Mayo Clinic. September 6, 2017. https://www.mayoclinic.org/healthy-lifestyle/nutrition-and-healthy-eating/in-depth/water/art-20044256.

Mayo Clinic Staff. 2018. 'Exercise and Stress: Get Moving to Manage Stress'. Mayo Clinic. March 8, 2018. https://www.mayoclinic.org/healthy-lifestyle/stress-management/in-depth/exercise-and-stress/art-20044469.

Mayo Clinic Staff. 2019. 'Omega-3 in Fish: How Eating Fish Helps Your Heart'. Mayo Clinic. September 28, 2019. http://www.mayoclinic.org/diseases-conditions/heart-disease/in-depth/omega-3/art-20045614.

McGroarty, B. 2018. 'Wellness Now a $4.2 Trillion Global Industry'. Global Wellness Institute. October 6, 2018. https://globalwellnessinstitute.org/press-room/press-releases/wellness-now-a-4-2-trillion-global-industry/.

Menon, V. P., and A. R. Sudheer. 2007. 'Antioxidant and Anti-inflammatory Properties of Curcumin'. In *The Molecular Targets and Therapeutic Uses of Curcumin in Health and Disease*, edited by B. B. Aggarwal, Y. J. Surh, and S. Shishodia, 105–25. Advances in Experimental Medicine and Biology 595. Boston: Springer. https://doi.org/10.1007/978-0-387-46401-5_3.

*Merriam-Webster's Collegiate Dictionary*, 11th ed. 2003. S.v. "willpower." Springfield, MA: Merriam-Webster.

Meyer, J. D., K. F. Koltyn, A. J. Stegner, J. Kim, and D. B. Cook. 2016. 'Influence of Exercise Intensity for Improving Depressed Mood in Depression: A Dose-Response Study'. *Behavior Therapy* 47, no. 4 (July): 527–37. https://doi.org/10.1016/j.beth.2016.04.003.

Mishra, S., and K. Palanivelu. 2008. 'The Effect of Curcumin (Turmeric) on Alzheimer's Disease: An Overview'. *Annals of Indian Academy of Neurology* 11, no. 1 (March): 13–19. https://doi.org/10.4103/0972-2327.40220.

Montgomery. P., J. R. Burton, R. P. Sewell. T. F. Spreckelsen, and A. J. Richardson. 2014. 'Fatty Acids and Sleep in UK Children: Subjective and Pilot Objective Sleep Results from the DOLAB Study—A Randomized Controlled Trial'. *Journal of Sleep Research* 23, no. 4 (August): 364–88. https://doi.org/10.1111/jsr.12135.

Morais, J. A., S. Chevalier, and R. Gougeon. 2006. 'Protein Turnover and Requirements in the Healthy and Frail Elderly'. *The Journal of Nutrition, Health & Aging* 10, no. 4 (August): 272–83.

Mozaffarian, D., I. Rosenberg, and R. Uauy. 2018. 'History of Modern Nutrition Science-Implications for Current Research, Dietary Guidelines, and Food Policy'. *BMJ* 361, no. k2392 (June). https://doi.org/10.1136/bmj.k2392.

Müller, M. J., A. Bosy-Westphal, and S. B. Heymsfield. 2010. 'Is There Evidence for a Set Point That Regulates Human Body Weight?' *F1000 Medicine Reports* 2, no. 59 (August). https://doi.org/10.3410/M2-59.

Murakami, K., S. Sasaki, H. Okubo, Y. Takahashi, Y. Hosoi, M. Itabashi, and Freshmen in Dietetic Courses Study Group II. 2007. 'Association Between Dietary Fiber, Water and Magnesium Intake and Functional Constipation Among Young Japanese Women'. *European Journal of Clinical Nutrition* 61, no. 5 (May): 616–22. https://doi.org/10.1038/sj.ejcn.1602573.

Murray, B. 2007. 'Hydration and Physical Performance'. *Journal of the American College of Nutrition* 26 (sup5: ILSI North America Conference on Hydration and Health): 542S–48S. https://doi.org/10.1080/07315724.2007.10719656.

Nagma, S., G. Kapoor, R. Bharti, A. Batra, A. Batra, A. Aggarwal, and A. Sablok. 2015. 'To Evaluate the Effect of Perceived Stress on Menstrual Function'. *JCDR* 9, no. 3 (March): QC01–QC03. https://doi.org/10.7860/JCDR/2015/6906.5611.

Nagpal, M., and S. Sood. 2013. 'Role of Curcumin in Systemic and Oral Health: An Overview'. *Journal of Natural Science, Biology, and Medicine* 4, no. 1 (January): 3–7. https://doi.org/10.4103/0976-9668.107253.

Nantz, M. P., C. A. Rowe, C. E. Muller, R. A. Creasy, J. M. Stanilka, and S. S. Percival. 2012. 'Supplementation With Aged Garlic Extract Improves Both NK and -T Cell Function and Reduces the Severity of Cold and Flu Symptoms: A Randomized, Double-Blind, Placebo-Controlled Nutrition Intervention'. *Clinical Nutrition* 31, no. 3 (June): 337–44. https://doi.org/10.1016/j.clnu.2011.11.019.

Nestle, M. 2001. 'Food Company Sponsorship of Nutrition Research and Professional Activities: A Conflict of Interest?' *Public Health Nutrition* 4, no. 5 (October): 1015–22. https://doi.org/10.1079/PHN2001253.

National Sleep Foundation. n.d. 'What is Healthy Sleep?' National Sleep Foundation Sleep Topics. Accessed [Febraury] [20], [2020]. https://www.sleepfoundation.org/articles/what-healthy-sleep.

NHS (National Health Service). 2017. 'Five-a-Day of Fruit and Veg Is Good, But "10 Is Better" '. NHS News. February 23, 2017. https://www.nhs.uk/news/food-and-diet/five-a-day-of-fruit-and-veg-is-good-but-10-is-better/.

———. 2018. 'Fish and Shellfish'. NHS Eat Well. Last reviewed December 4, 2018. https://www.nhs.uk/live-well/eat-well/fish-and-shellfish-nutrition/.

———. 2020. 'Stress'. https://www.mayoclinic.org/healthy-lifestyle/stress-management/in-depth/stress-symptoms/art-20050987

Obert, J., M. Pearlman, L. Obert, and S. Chapin. 2017. 'Popular Weight Loss Strategies: A Review of Four Weight Loss Techniques'. *Current Gastroenterology Reports* 19, no. 61 (November). https://doi.org/10.1007/s11894-017-0603-8.

O' Donovan, F., S. Carney, J. Kennedy, H. Hayes, N. Pender, F. Boland, and A. Stanton. 2019. 'Associations and Effects of Omega-3 Polyunsaturated Fatty Acids on Cognitive Function and Mood in Healthy Adults: A Protocol for a Systematic Review of Observational and Interventional Studies'. *BMJ Open* 9, no. 6 (June): e027167. https://doi.org/10.1136/bmjopen-2018-027167.

Owen, R. W., A. Giacosa, W. E. Hull, R. Haubner, B. Spiegelhalder, and H. Bartsch. 2000. 'The Antioxidant/Anticancer Potential of Phenolic Compounds Isolated From Olive Oil. *European Journal of Cancer* 36, no. 10 (June): 1235–47. https://doi.org/10.1016/s0959-8049(00)00103-9.

Owen, R. W., R. Haubner, G. Würtele, W. E. Hull, B. Spiegelhalder, and H. Bartsch. 2004. 'Olives and Olive Oil in Cancer Prevention'. *European Journal of Cancer Prevention*, 13, no. 4 (August): 319–26. https://doi.org/10.1097/01.cej.0000130221.19480.7e.

Palascha, A., E. van Kleef, and H. C. M. van Trijp. 2015. 'How Does Thinking in Black and White Terms Relate to Eating Behavior and Weight Regain?' *Journal of Health Psychology* 20, no. 5 (May): 638–48. https://doi.org/10.1177/1359105315573440.

Passey, C. 2017. 'Reducing the Dietary Acid Load: How a More Alkaline Diet Benefits Patients With Chronic Kidney Disease'. *Journal of Renal Nutrition* 27, no. 3 (May): 151–60. https://doi.org/10.1053/j.jrn.2016.11.006.

Patel, S. R., and F. B. Hu. 2008. 'Short Sleep Duration and Weight Gain: A Systematic Review'. *Obesity* 16, no. 3 (March): 643–53. https://doi.org/10.1038/oby.2007.118.

Patterson, R. E., G. A. Laughlin, A. Z. LaCroix, S. J. Hartman, L. Natarajan, C. M. Senger, M. E. Martínez, A. Villaseñor, D. D. Sears, C. R. Marinac, and L. C. Gallo. 2015. 'Intermittent Fasting and Human Metabolic Health'. *Journal of the Academy of Nutrition and Dietetics* 115, no. 8 (August): 1203–12. https://doi.org/10.1016/j.jand.2015.02.018.

Payne, C., P. J. Wiffen, and S. Martin. 2012. 'Interventions for Fatigue and Weight Loss in Adults With Advanced Progressive Illness'. *The Cochrane Database of Systematic Reviews* 1, no. CD008427 (January). https://doi.org/10.1002/14651858.CD008427.pub2.

Pedrinolla, A., F. Schena, and M. Venturelli. 2017. 'Resilience to Alzheimer's Disease: The Role of Physical Activity'. *Current Alzheimer Research* 14 (5): 546–53. https://doi.org/10.2174/1567205014666170111145817.

Pham, A. Q., H. Kourlas, and D. Q. Pham. 2007. 'Cinnamon Supplementation in Patients With Type 2 Diabetes Mellitus'. *Pharmacotherapy* 27, no. 4 (April): 595–99. https://doi.org/10.1592/phco.27.4.595.

Pistollato, F., S. Sumalla Cano, I. Elio, M. Masias Vergara, F. Giampieri, and M. Battino. 2016. 'Associations Between Sleep, Cortisol Regulation, and Diet: Possible Implications for the Risk of Alzheimer Disease'. *Advances in Nutrition* 7, no. 4 (July): 679–89. https://doi.org/10.3945/an.115.011775.

Polheber, J. P., and R. L. Matchock. 2014. 'The Presence of a Dog Attenuates Cortisol and Heart Rate in the Trier Social Stress Test Compared to Human Friends'. *Journal of Behavioral Medicine* 37, no. 5 (October): 860–67. https://doi.org/10.1007/s10865-013-9546-1.

Popkin, B. M., K. E. D'Anci, and I. H. Rosenberg. 2010. 'Water, Hydration, and Health'. *Nutrition Reviews* 68, no. 8 (August): 439–58. https://doi.org/10.1111/j.1753-4887.2010.00304.x.

Powell, D. J. H., C. Liossi, R. Moss-Morris, and W. Schlotz. 2013. 'Unstimulated Cortisol Secretory Activity in Everyday Life and Its Relationship With Fatigue and Chronic Fatigue Syndrome: A Systematic Review and Subset Meta-analysis'. *Psychoneuroendocrinology* 38, no. 11 (November): 2405–22. https://doi.org/10.1016/j.psyneuen.2013.07.004.

Pross, N., A. Demazieres, N. Girard, R. Barnouin, F. Santoro, E. Chevillotte, A. Klein, and L. Le Bellego. 2013. 'Influence of Progressive Fluid Restriction on Mood and Physiological Markers of Dehydration in Women'. *British Journal of Nutrition* 109, no. 2 (January): 313–21. https://doi.org/10.1017/S0007114512001080.

Public Health England. 2018. 'PHE Publishes Latest Data on Nation's Diet'. United Kingdom Government Press Release. March 16, 2018. https://www.gov.uk/government/news/phe-publishes-latest-data-on-nations-diet.

Puetz, T. W. 2006. 'Physical Activity and Feelings of Energy and Fatigue: Epidemiological Evidence'. *Sports Medicine* 36, no. 9 (September): 767–80. https://doi.org/10.2165/00007256-200636090-00004.

Pulido, R., M. Hernandez-Garcia, and F. Saura-Calixto. 2003. 'Contribution of Beverages to the Intake of Lipophilic and Hydrophilic Antioxidants in the Spanish Diet'. *European Journal of Clinical Nutrition* 57, no. 10 (October): 1275–82. https://doi.org/10.1038/sj.ejcn.1601685.

Qin, B., K. S. Panickar, and R. A. Anderson. 2010. 'Cinnamon: Potential Role in the Prevention of Insulin Resistance, Metabolic Syndrome, and Type 2 Diabetes'. *Journal of Diabetes Science and Technology* 4, no. 3 (May): 685–93. https://doi.org/10.1177/193229681000400324.

Reilly, N. R. 2016. 'The Gluten-Free Diet: Recognizing Fact, Fiction, and Fad'. *Journal of Pediatrics* 175 (August): 206–10. https://doi.org/10.1016/j.jpeds.2016.04.014.

Research and Markets. 2019. 'The U.S. Weight Loss and Diet Control Market'. https://www.researchandmarkets.com/research/qm2gts/the_72_billion?w=4.

Riley, K. E., and C. L. Park. 2015. 'How Does Yoga Reduce Stress? A Systematic Review of Mechanisms of Change and Guide to Future Inquiry'. *Health Psychology Review* 9 (3), 379–96. https://doi.org/10.1080/17437199.2014.981778.

Rivlin, R. S. 2001. 'Historical Perspective on the Use of Garlic'. *The Journal of Nutrition* 131, no. 3 (March): 951S-54S. https://doi.org/10.1093/jn/131.3.951S.

Roepe, L. R. 2018. The Diet Industry. Sage Business Researcher. March 5, 2018. http://businessresearcher.sagepub.com/sbr-1946-105904-2881576/20180305/the-diet-industry.

Rynders, C. A., E. A. Thomas, A. Zaman, Z. Pan, V. A. Catenacci, and E. L. Melanson. 2019. 'Effectiveness of Intermittent Fasting and Time-Restricted Feeding Compared to Continuous Energy Restriction for Weight Loss'. *Nutrients* 11, no. 10 (October): 2442. https://doi.org/10.3390/nu11102442.

Schaefer, J. T., and A. B. Magnuson. 2014. 'A Review of Interventions That Promote Eating by Internal Cues'. Journal of the Academy of Nutrition and Dietetics 114, no. 5 (May): 734–60. https://doi.org/10.1016/j.jand.2013.12.024.

Schwalfenberg, G. K. 2012. 'The Alkaline Diet: Is There Evidence That an Alkaline pH Diet Benefits Health?' *Journal of Environmental and Public Health* 2012 (727630). https://doi.org/10.1155/2012/727630.

Seid, H., and M. Rosenbaum. 2019. 'Low Carbohydrate and Low-Fat Diets: What We Don't Know and Why We Should Know It'. *Nutrients* 11, no. 11 (November): 2749. https://doi.org/10.3390/nu11112749.

Serrur, M. 2017. 'The Most Popular Diets of Every Decade Since 1900 Slideshow 1900s'. The Daily Meal. April 18, 2017. https://www.thedailymeal.com/healthy-eating/most-popular-diets-every-decade-1900-slideshow.

Shan, B., Y. Z. Cai, M. Sun, and H. Corke. 2005. 'Antioxidant Capacity of 26 Spice Extracts and Characterization of Their Phenolic Constituents'. *Journal of Agricultural and Food Chemistry* 53, no. 20 (October): 7749–59. https://doi.org/10.1021/jf051513y.

Simpson, H. L., and B. J. Campbell. 2015. 'Review Article: Dietary Fibre-Microbiota Interactions'. *Alimentary Pharmacology and Therapeutics* 42, no. 2 (July): 158–79. https://doi.org/10.1111/apt.13248.

Slentz, C. A., J. A. Houmard, and W. E. Kraus. 2009. 'Exercise, Abdominal Obesity, Skeletal Muscle, and Metabolic Risk: Evidence for a Dose Response'. *Obesity* 17, no. S3 (December): S27–S33. https://doi.org/10.1038/oby.2009.385.

SlimFast. n.d. 'Slim Fast: Our Story'. About Us. Accessed [January] [25], 2020. https://www.slimfast.co.uk/about-us.

Smith, A. P., P. Brockman, R. Flynn, A. Maben, and M. Thomas. 1993. 'Investigation of the Effects of Coffee on Alertness and Performance During the Day and Night'. *Neuropsychobiology* 27 (4): 217–23. https://doi.org/10.1159/000118984.

Sobenin, I. A., I. V. Andrianova, O. N. Demidova, T. Gorchakova, and A. N. Orekhov. 2008. 'Lipid-Lowering Effects of Time-Released Garlic Powder Tablets in Double-Blinded Placebo-Controlled Randomized Study'. *Journal of Atherosclerosis and Thrombosis* 15, no. 6 (December): 334–38. https://doi.org/10.5551/jat.e550.

Sorkin, B. C., A. J. Kuszak, J. S. Williamson, D. C. Hopp, and J. M. Betz. 2016. 'The Challenge of Reproducibility and Accuracy in Nutrition Research: Resources and Pitfalls'. *Advances in Nutrition* 7, no. 2 (March): 383–89. https://doi.org/10.3945/an.115.010595.

Steptoe, A., S. Dockray, and J. Wardle. 2009. 'Positive Affect and Psychobiological Processes Relevant to Health'. *Journal of Personality* 77, no. 6 (December): 1747–76. https://doi.org/10.1111/j.1467-6494.2009.00599.x.

Stice, E., and K. Burger. 2015. 'Dieting as a Risk Factor for Eating Disorders'. In *The Wiley Handbook of Eating Disorders*, edited by L. Smolak and M. P. Levine, 312–23. https://doi.org/doi:10.1002/9781118574089.ch24.

Stice, E., J. M. Gau, P. Rohde, and H. Shaw. 2017. 'Risk Factors That Predict Future Onset of Each DSM-5 Eating Disorder: Predictive Specificity in High-Risk Adolescent Females'. *Journal of Abnormal Psychology* 126, no. 1 (January): 38–51. https://doi.org/10.1037/abn0000219.

Sutherland, J., M. Miles, D. Hedderley, J. Li, S. Devoy, K. Sutton, and D. Lauren. 2009. 'In Vitro Effects of Food Extracts on Selected Probiotic and Pathogenic Bacteria'. *International Journal of Food Sciences and Nutrition* 60 (8): 717–27. https://doi.org/https://dx.doi.org/10.3109/09637480802165650.

Sweeney, M. E., J. O. Hill, P. A. Heller, R. Baney, and M. DiGirolamo. 1993. 'Severe vs Moderate Energy Restriction With and Without Exercise in the Treatment of Obesity: Efficiency of Weight Loss'. *American Journal of Clinical Nutrition* 57, no. 2 (February): 127–34. https://doi.org/10.1093/ajcn/57.2.127.

Tipton, K. D., and R. R. Wolfe. 2001. 'Exercise, Protein Metabolism, and Muscle Growth'. *International Journal of Sport Nutrition and Exercise Metabolism* 11, no. 1 (March): 109–32. https://doi.org/10.1123/ijsnem.11.1.109.

Tobey, J. A. 1936. 'The Question of Acid and Alkali Forming Foods'. *American Journal of Public Health* 26, no. 11 (November): 1113–16. https://doi.org/10.2105/ajph.26.11.1113.

Tobias, D. K., M. Chen, J. E. Manson, D. S. Ludwig, W. Willett, and F. B. Hu. 2015. 'Effect of Low-Fat Diet Interventions Versus Other Diet Interventions on Long-Term Weight Change in Adults: A Systematic Review and Meta-analysis'. *The Lancet Diabetes & Endocrinology* 3, no. 12 (December): 968–79. https://doi.org/10.1016/S2213-8587(15)00367-8.

Tribole, E., and E. Resch. 1996. *Intuitive Eating*. New York: St. Martin's Paperbacks.

Trichopoulou, A., P. Lagiou, H. Kuper, and D. Trichopoulos. 2000. 'Cancer and Mediterranean Dietary Traditions'. *Cancer Epidemiology, Biomarkers & Prevention* 9, no. 9 (September): 869–73.

Turan, B., C. Foltz, J. F. Cavanagh, B. A. Wallace, M. Cullen, E. L. Rosenberg, P. A. Jennings, P. Ekman, and M. E. Kemeny. 2015. 'Anticipatory Sensitization to Repeated Stressors: The Role of Initial Cortisol Reactivity and Meditation/Emotion Skills Training'. *Psychoneuroendocrinology* 52 (February): 229–38. https://doi.org/10.1016/j.psyneuen.2014.11.014.

Uedo, N., H. Ishikawa, K. Morimoto, R. Ishihara, H. Narahara, I. Akedo, T. Ioka, I. Kaji, and S. Fukuda. 2004. 'Reduction in Salivary Cortisol Level by Music Therapy During Colonoscopic Examination'. *Hepato-Gastroenterology* 51, no. 56 (March): 451–53.

Vahia, V. N. 2013. 'Diagnostic and Statistical Manual of Mental Disorders 5: A Quick Glance'. *Indian Journal of Psychiatry* 55, no. 3 (July–September): 220–23. https://doi.org/10.4103/0019-5545.117131.

Van Dyke, N., and E. J. Drinkwater. 2014. 'Relationships Between Intuitive Eating and Health Indicators: Literature Review'. *Public Health Nutrition* 17, no. 8 (August): 1757–66. https://doi.org/10.1017/S1368980013002139.

Varga, M., S. Dukay-Szabó, F. Túry, and F. van Furth Eric. 2013. 'Evidence and Gaps in the Literature on Orthorexia Nervosa'. *Eating and Weight Disorders* 18, no. 2 (June): 103–11. https://doi.org/10.1007/s40519-013-0026-y.

Vicennati, V., F. Pasqui, C. Cavazza, U. Pagotto, and R. Pasquali. 2009. 'Stress-Related Development of Obesity and Cortisol in Women'. *Obesity* 17, no. 9 (September): 1678–83. https://doi.org/10.1038/oby.2009.76.

Wagner, C. 2019. 'Are Mexican Avocados the Next "Conflct Commodity"?' Verisk Maplecroft. December 5, 2019. https://www.maplecroft.com/insights/analysis/are-mexican-avocados-the-next-conflict-commodity/.

Walton, K., L. Kuczynski, E. Haycraft, A. Breen, and J. Haines. 2017. 'Time to Re-think Picky Eating?: A Relational Approach to Understanding Picky Eating'. *International Journal of Behavioral Nutrition and Physical Activity* 14 (62). https://doi.org/10.1186/s12966-017-0520-0.

Weaver, C. M., and J. W. Miller. 2017. 'Challenges in Conducting Clinical Nutrition Research'. *Nutrition Reviews* 75, no. 7 (July): 491–99. https://doi.org/10.1093/nutrit/nux026.

Weight Watchers. n.d. 'History and Philosophy'. About Us. Accessed [February] [2], 2020. https://www.weightwatchers.com/about/his/history.aspx.

Wienecke, E., and C. Nolden. 2016. 'Long-Term HRV Analysis Shows Stress Reduction by Magnesium Intake'. *MMW* 158, no. S6 (December), 12–16. https://doi.org/10.1007/s15006-016-9054-7.

Willett, W., J. Rockstrom, B. Loken, M. Springmann, T. Lang, S. Vermeulen, T. Garnett et al. 2019. 'Food in the Anthropocene: The EAT-*Lancet* Commission on Healthy Diets From Sustainable Food Systems'. *Lancet* 393, no. 10170 (February): 447–92. https://doi.org/10.1016/S0140-6736(18)31788-4.

Winston, A. P., E. Hardwick, and N. Jaberi. 2005. 'Neuropsychiatric Effects of Caffeine'. *Advances in Psychiatric Treatment* 11, no. 6 (November): 432–39. https://doi.org/DOI: 10.1192/apt.11.6.432.

Wolpert, S. 2007. 'Dieting Does Not Work, UCLA Researchers Report'. UCLA Newsroom. April 3, 2007. https://newsroom.ucla.edu/releases/Dieting-Does-Not-Work-UCLA-Researchers-7832.

World Health Organization. 2018. 'A Healthy Diet Sustainably Produced'. Information Sheet. November 2018. https://apps.who.int/iris/bitstream/handle/10665/278948/WHO-NMH-NHD-18.12-eng.pdf?ua=1.

Yu, L. 2019. 'Superfoods' Dark Side: Increasing Vulnerability of Quinoa Farmers in Bolivia'. Colby College. January 22, 2019. http://web.colby.edu/st297-global18/2019/0½2/superfoods-dark-side-increasing-vulnerability-of-quinoa-farmers-in-bolivia/.

Zendegui, E. A., J. A. West, and L. J. Zandberg. 2014. 'Binge Eating Frequency and Regular Eating Adherence: The Role of Eating Pattern in Cognitive Behavioral Guided Self-help'. *Eating Behaviors* 15, no. 2 (April): 241–43. https://doi.org/10.1016/j.eatbeh.2014.03.002.

Zhong, V. W., L. Van Horn, M. C. Cornelis, J. T. Wilkins, H. Ning, M. R. Carnethon, P. Greenland et al. 2019. 'Associations of Dietary Cholesterol or Egg Consumption With Incident Cardiovascular Disease and Mortality'. *JAMA* 321, no. 11 (March): 1081–95. https://doi.org/10.1001/jama.2019.1572.

Zulfarina, M. S., A. M. Sharkawi, Z. Aqilah-S. N., S. Mokhtar, S. A. Nazrun, and I. Naina-Mohamed, I. 2016. 'Influence of Adolescents' Physical Activity on Bone Mineral Acquisition: A Systematic Review Article'. *Iranian Journal of Public Health* 45, no. 12 (December): 1545–57.

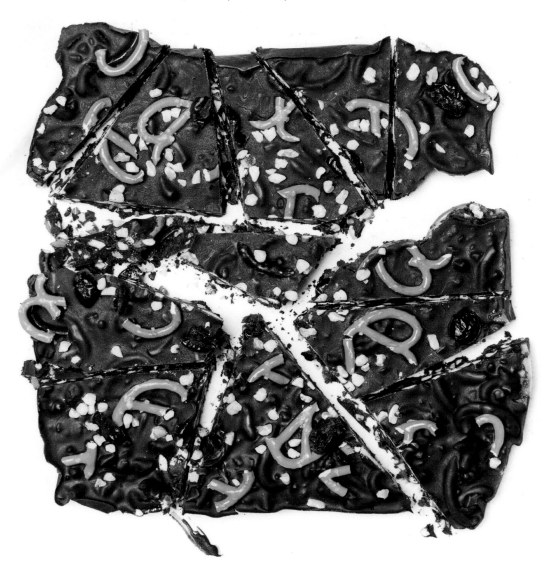

# Acknowledgments

We are so grateful to have been given the opportunity to write a book together. As nutrition professionals, we think it's so important to spread a positive and realistic message that will reach as many people as possible. We hope this book will be a helpful tool for so many.

Thank you to Meyer and Meyer for believing we had something important enough to say, and thank you to Liz Evans who worked closely with us to bring this to life.

We are eternally grateful for our 'Forking Wellness' podcast community! Thank you, guys, for tuning in each week and ultimately allowing us to grow as a brand! This would not be possible without you all.

Thank you to our lovely friend and photographer, Lizzy Clough, for capturing such beautiful shots of both us and our recipes, and to Gemma Fee for our hair and make-up.

We have both had a challenging journey with regard to making it to this point and would like to thank some significant people in our lives individually...

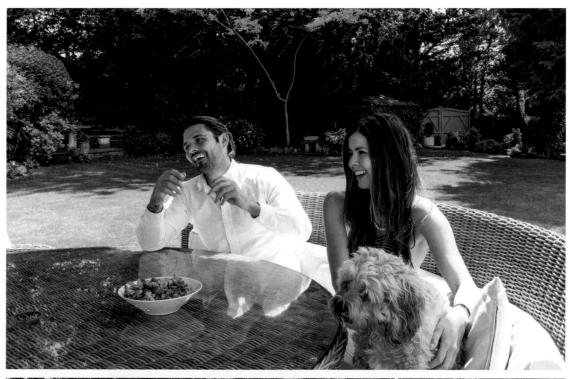

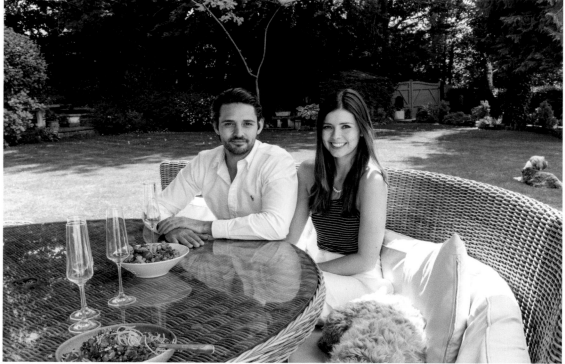

I would not be where I am today without the incredible and ongoing support from my family. I cannot express how grateful I am to have such loving and understanding parents who have always been there to guide and encourage me to believe in myself no matter what. Thank you to my sister Kitty, twin brothers Tom and James, my Nana and Grandma, and friends Saskia, Emma, Rob, Katie, Georgie, Rhiannon, and Bari for being a part of my amazing support system!

My gorgeous husband Ash always said he could see me on the front cover of my own book one day... he called it! Thank you, Ash, for being such a loving and positive person to live life with. I love you so much.

–Sophie

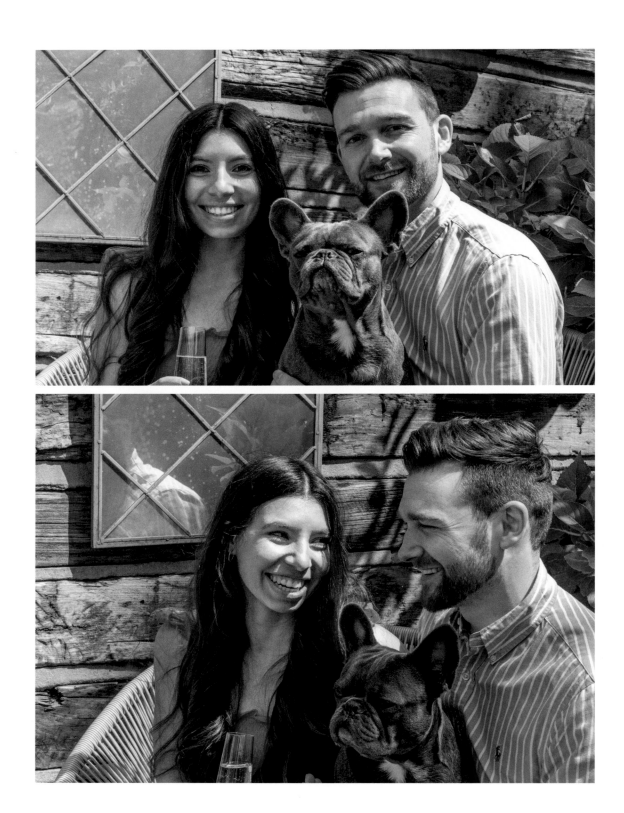

I want to thank my entire family as well. Even from across the pond, you've all continued to encourage me, believe in me, and unconditionally support me. To Fran, Alan, Josh, Grandma Gloria, Grandma Judy, and Poppy Marvin—thank you for always being there for me, no matter what!

To my friends, both in the UK and America, I feel beyond lucky to have you all! From Delaware to NYC, London to Sevenoaks, I am incredibly grateful. And of course, thank you to Sophie for being a dream co-author, best friend, and podcast host!

Lastly, a big thank you to my partner Mark for being my number 1 fan, my cheerleader, and my rock. Thanks for always being there for me and pushing me to be the best version of myself.

*−Bari*

# Recipe Index

# Conversion Charts

| Dry Weights | |
|---|---|
| Metric | Imperial |
| 5g | ¼ oz |
| 8/10g | ⅓ oz |
| 15g | ½ oz |
| 20g | ¾ oz |
| 25g | 1oz |
| 30/35g | 1¼ oz |
| 40g | 1 ½ oz |
| 50g | 2 oz |
| 60/70g | 2 ½ oz |
| 75/85/90g | 3 oz |
| 100g | 3 ½ oz |
| 110/120g | 4 oz |
| 125/130g | 4 ½ oz |
| 135/140/150g | 5oz |
| 170/175g | 6oz |
| 200g | 7oz |
| 225g | 8oz |
| 250g | 9oz |
| 265g | 9 ½ oz |
| 275g | 10oz |

| | |
|---|---|
| 300g | 11oz |
| 325g | 11 ½ oz |
| 350g | 12oz |
| 375g | 13oz |
| 400g | 14oz |
| 425g | 15oz |
| 450g | 1lb |
| 475g | 1lb. 1oz |
| 500g | 1lb. 2oz |
| 550g | 1lb. 3oz |
| 600g | 1lb. 5oz |
| 625g | 1lb. 6oz |
| 650g | 1lb. 7oz |
| 675g | 1 ½ lb |
| 700g | 1lb. 9oz |
| 750g | 1lb 10oz |
| 800g | 1 ¾ lb |
| 850g | 1lb. 14oz |
| 900g | 2lb. |
| 950g | 2lb. 2oz |
| 1kg | 2lb. 3oz |

| Liquid Measurements | | |
|---|---|---|
| Metric | Imperial | Cups |
| 15ml | ½ fl oz | 1 tbsp (level) |
| 20ml | ¾ fl oz | |
| 25ml | 1 fl oz | ⅛ cup |
| 30ml | 1 ¼ fl oz | |
| 50ml | 2 fl oz | ¼ cup |
| 60ml | 2 ½ fl oz | |
| 75ml | 3 fl oz | |
| 100ml | 3 ½ fl oz | ⅜ cup |
| 110/120ml | 4 fl oz | ½ cup |
| 125ml | 4 ½ fl oz | |
| 150ml | 5 fl oz | ⅔ cup |
| 175ml | 6 fl oz | ¾ cup |
| 200/215ml | 7 fl oz | |
| 225ml | 8 fl oz | 1 cup |
| 250ml | 9 fl oz | |
| 275ml | 9 ½ fl oz | |
| 300ml | ½ pint | 1 ¼ cups |
| 350ml | 12 fl oz | 1 ½ cups |
| 375ml | 13 fl oz | |
| 400ml | 14 fl oz | |
| 425ml | 15 fl oz | |
| 450ml | 16 fl oz | 2 cups |
| 500ml | 18 fl oz | 2 ¼ cups |
| 550ml | 19 fl oz | |
| 600ml | 1 pint | 2 ½ cups |
| 700ml | 1 ¼ pints | |

| | | |
|---|---|---|
| 750ml | 1 ⅓ pints | |
| 800ml | 1 pint, 9 fl oz | |
| 850ml | 1 ½ pints | |
| 900ml | 1 pint, 12 fl oz | 3 ¾ cups |
| 1 litre | 1 ¾ pints | 4 cups |

| Oven Temperatures* | | |
|---|---|---|
| °C | °F | Gas Mark |
| 110 | 225 | ¼ |
| 130 | 250 | ½ |
| 140 | 275 | 1 |
| 150 | 300 | 2 |
| 160/170 | 325 | 3 |
| 180 | 350 | 4 |
| 190 | 375 | 5 |
| 200 | 400 | 6 |
| 220 | 425 | 7 |
| 230 | 450 | 8 |
| 240 | 475 | 9 |

*The temperatures indicated in the recipes are all based on using a fan-assisted oven. If you are using a conventional oven, increase the temperature by 20°C.

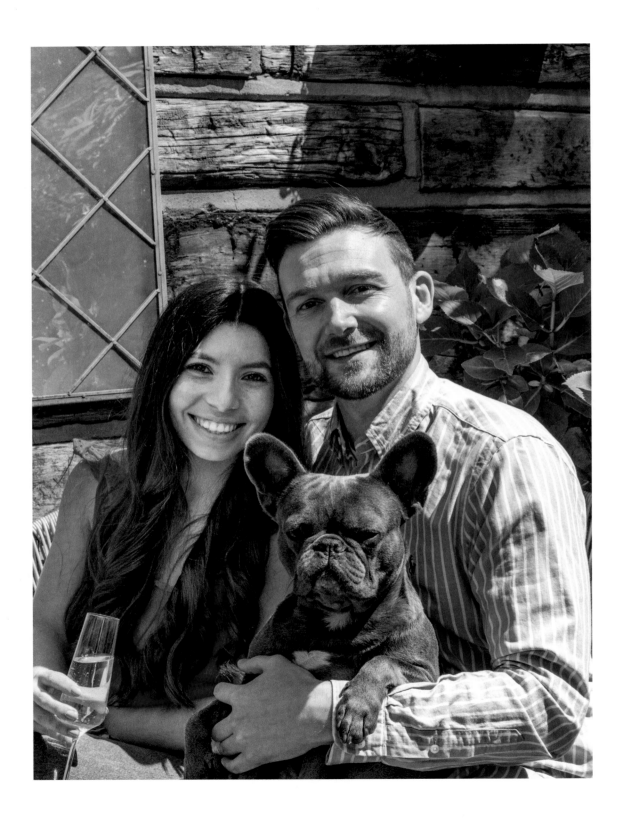

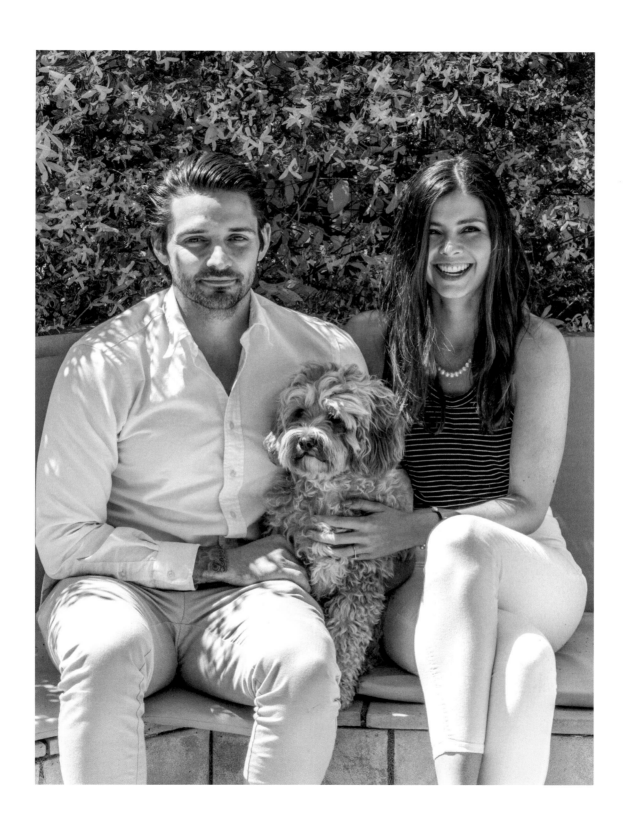

# Credits

**Cover and interior design:** Annika Naas

**Layout:** Guido Maetzing, www.mmedia-agentur.de

**Cover and interior photos:** © Meyer & Meyer Sport (UK) Ltd.

**Photographer:** Lizzy Rose Clough, www.lizzyroseclough.com

**Managing editor:** Elizabeth Evans